The Ultimate Guide
to Fellatio

Ultimate Guides from Cleis Press

The Ultimate Guide to Anal Sex for Men
by Bill Brent

The Ultimate Guide to Anal Sex for Women
by Tristan Taormino

The Ultimate Guide to Cunnilingus
by Violet Blue

The Ultimate Guide to Pregnancy for Lesbians
by Rachel Pepper

The Ultimate Guide to Strap-on Sex
by Karlyn Lotney

The Ultimate Guide to Fellatio

How to Go Down on a Man
and Give Him Mind-Blowing Pleasure

VIOLET BLUE

CLEIS
PRESS

Published in the United States by Cleis Press Inc., P.O. Box 14684, San Francisco, California 94114.

Printed in the United States.
Cover design: Scott Idleman
Book design: Karen Quigg
Cleis Press logo art: Juana Alicia
First Edition.
10 9 8 7 6 5 4

Acknowledgments

When writing a sex book, it's easy to feel like you're alone on an island of research and data, syntax and smut. But not in this case—this book contains the voices of (literally) hundreds of people who responded to postings, queries, and a questionnaire. People who loaned me their personal stories and quotes, helped me find essential information, and tipped me off to resources. Thank you.

If sex books are islands, then the Cleis empire supplies the life rafts. Felice Newman, source of unending support, advice, humor, and delightful enthusiasm for sex education, thank you for your incredible help and willingness to roll up your sleeves and dig—for answers or for solutions. Don, I live to bug you. Thank you for your patience, sweetness, charm, and kind words. Frédérique, your smiles buoy me, and your commitment to your passions inspires me. Thanks, Cleis.

On my little fellatio island, I had many visitors. Constance Clare, thank you for all of your laughter and silly, silly jokes, and your total faith in me over the years. Family is important, and mine is big, scary, hilarious, and strong: thank you to my close-knit community of Survival Research Laboratories. We did an amazing show in the middle of my writing this dirty, dirty book, and without your support and friendship I would certainly have had a record-breaking personality meltdown. Mark, thank you for the love, merciless teasing, bottomless friendship, tireless support, and for clearing me a place at SRL to burn the midnight oil on this manuscript. Michael S., thanks for listening.

Thomas Roche, my dear friend, thank you forever! Not only did you lend your considerable knowledge as a SFSI instructor and highly polished eye to this text, but you also tirelessly talked shop with me whenever I needed it, sometimes very late at night. Thanks to Cara Bruce, brilliant woman that you are, for the last-minute support and the schemes, and the deep friendship. Jenny Morse, you tasty morsel, thank you for helping me in the ways a girl can help another girl do research on books about giving head. You're naughty and the best. Alex, I followed all your suggestions, thank you. And Courtney—my tireless research assistant—thanks for the rug burn, my love.

This little time capsule wouldn't be complete without thanking my closest friend, Todd. Our connection, the endurance of our friendship, the belief you have in me—all these things mean the world to me. You helped me in so many ways. I can't thank you enough.

Contents

Illustrations

Foreword

It's difficult for me to hide my enthusiasm for fellatio. At first glance it seems like such a straightforward sex act, but when you look closely, it's actually quite versatile. There are innumerable ways for me to enjoy how I give it, how my partner receives it, and how I choose to receive it myself (think the business end of a strap-on). There's the pure pleasure of taking my lover into my mouth for the sole concentrated purpose of giving him direct, focused gratification. My intentions when giving head are concrete: oral contact, mouth to cock, an immediate sensation that clearly sends him the message that I want to give him pleasure, now. The feelings of not only having my lover's delicate genitals in my mouth but also being able to directly control his stimulation are intoxicating. The primal sensory information of taking in the essence, taste, smell, and outrageously sexy up-close visuals of my lover is a powerful aphrodisiac that influences me physically, mentally, emotionally, and on levels I believe I simply cannot detect. And it's an undeniable fact that my mouth is a sex organ. The moment I've got my lover in my mouth, the heat of desire, passion, and lust in focus, right in front of me, ties my arousal directly to him.

The ways I can elicit my own arousal from fellatio are endless: Giving head works itself easily into any context or scenario I can dream up. My fantasies make anything possible, and these fantasies can be accelerated by the mere fact that fellatio can be performed almost anywhere. I can be a dominant woman, doling out pleasure as I see fit—or I can even be a naughty young man with a pretty mouth. I can play with roles, becoming an overly dedicated nurse for a helpless patient, an earnest applicant for an important job, or a submissive slave. The exchange can be an act of love, tenderness, and devotion, and gazing into my partner's eyes I can revel in the emotion and sensuality of it all. Or together we can make it a filthy, wicked blow job; quick, dirty, and hot. Any way I choose to approach or experience fellatio, it's delightful. And I know I'm giving my lover powerful, focused pleasure.

My perspective on fellatio has been reshaped many times as I've had different experiences and relationships to oral sex. I didn't always like it. The first few times were difficult, confusing, and embarrassing. I wasn't sure what to do: I had a basic idea of how to perform the act, but I had no clue what my lovers might like, what I should be doing with my mouth, or how I should be feeling about the whole thing. What I now know is that the knowing smile and heated body language of a lover who wants oral sex was (back then) my dreaded cue to try to act experienced with my fumbling hands and tentative mouth. It felt like those dreams in which you go to class for a big exam and you're naked—I felt exposed and found myself wondering how I got there, and how the heck to get through it. I didn't know anything about the rhythm leading to orgasm, how a penis responds to pleasure—or worse, if I should be feeling humiliated by an act widely considered submissive, "easy," or demeaning. I'd gag and choke, and my eyes would water, and though my lovers enjoyed my enthusiasm to keep trying to make them feel good, I just felt lost and embarrassed.

Years passed, and I went through periods of giving up on trying to be good at fellatio, not knowing if I was any good at it, or if fellatio made me less worthy of respect by my partners. Even more confusing, I didn't know why giving head turned me on so much. Turns out I was normal, but not having much fun with fellatio.

Now, I'm a professional sex educator for Good Vibrations. My first year with them was spent working in the stores as a Sex Educator/Sales Associate, providing accurate sex information to hundreds of customers face-to-face. It's no easy feat to become an SESA for Good Vibes: there's a required twenty-one-hour training program, a comprehensive reading list, and quarterly continuing education classes. In my current position I write Good Vibes's educational materials (working closely with the Education and Outreach departments) and all the book and video reviews. I'm also a sex writer, penning columns about sex and sexuality for Web magazines. I have come full circle with my own experiences, and I am also in touch with other people's, and I have read and watched everything about oral sex I could find.

Writing this book was an enormous undertaking. I read and reread everything about fellatio, scoured sex guidebooks and modern erotica, and shook the Internet until it rattled. In addition, I received responses to questionnaires from over 150 people in the United States, Europe, and Canada, people who comprised the full spectrum of gender, sexual preference, age, race, and ability. I gathered their comments, compiled my research, and looked at the results with the sex-positive, nonjudgmental approach to sexuality that I learned at Good Vibrations.

All the people who responded to me have allowed me to quote them, and the text is liberally laced with their comments. I got a spectrum of responses to the subject matter—everything from excitement to disapproval. Everyone seemed to have something to say about fellatio, but most folks figured that it was the one-trick pony of sex with men. Men like it; you suck their cocks, it makes them come—simple. And it's just this oversimplification of sex—especially male sexuality—that keeps us confused and in the dark about men and pleasure.

Why is the subject of men and sexual pleasure so glossed over, reduced to "in and out"? Understanding how someone (male or female) enjoys sex goes much deeper than stereotypes. Whenever the subject of men and sex is written about, it's either predictably adolescent, cloaked and choked in New Age spiritualism, or clinically dry and sterile. No matter where you look, male sexuality is everywhere, and yet it is still presented as something to be ashamed of. What kind of choices are these?

When it comes to male sexual pleasure and fellatio, the terms become even more reduced to stereotypes, and the information is shallow. Popular magazines present tricks to "wow your fella," giving instant-gratification tips that help you do something just slightly titillating, without really telling you how to do anything related to the person whose body part you're

having sex with. The messages we get from the magazines, the media, and the people who perpetuate the
stereotypes about oral sex and guys is that head is all
guys want, that all guys want head, and that it's an easy
way to get them off—because guys are easy to get off.
How insulting. To say that these attitudes misrepresent
male sexuality is an understatement—and in their igno-
rance they interfere with our ability to have thoughtful,
hot, and effectively pleasurable oral sex with our male
partners.

The sex guides that are available are no better. Delve
into a book that covers fellatio, and you'll find a predictable slew of material that tells you what you can do
to your easily pleased man. But what you won't find is a
thorough, mindful investigation of men and sex—even
sex guidebooks written by men are circumspect. The
ones written for men are even more insulting, boiling sex
terms into bite-sized chunks of sports euphemisms, as if
they needed to "dumb down" the information into
simple, digestible terms that men can understand!

This "dumbing down" in virtually all the guidebooks
that cover male sexuality makes everything worse, per-
petuating the instant-gratification myths that men must
constantly cope with, and in an almost sinister way, hint-
ing at the author's own distaste for the material. It's as if
they wanted to get through it as quickly as possible—it
begs the question about the author's own comfort and
judgments about men and sex. Most of these books are
written from a heterosexual perspective, which makes
me wonder if it's a pervasive homophobia that causes
authors to recoil from the subject. I've come to believe
that including the gay perspective makes straight authors
nervous, as if fuzzing the neat little boxes they've put
men and women into would somehow ruin everything.
Perhaps, for them, it would. So when straight authors

cover fellatio, they do so quickly, they invent insulting names for techniques, and they never, ever get into the dirty details of how come tastes, or how to deep throat. They are also handicapped by a serious lack of understanding about male anatomy and how it responds to pleasure, and they omit or hurry through one important part of men's sexual anatomy: the anus and prostate. Clearly, to omit the gay male perspective leaves out a wealth of information—gay male experience, books, and videos are rich resources for all women and men.

Nothing was left out of this book. This is where you'll find everything you need to know to give incredible head, and more. This is where you'll get honest information about male pleasure. This is where you can crash the gates of sex play and learn how to go down on a strap-on dildo. This book fearlessly slashes stereotypes, treads into forbidden pleasure zones. It doesn't shy away from advanced techniques. Here is where you'll find everything the other books left out: anatomy for pleasure, genital massage, shaving, a complete investigation of deep-throat techniques, flavored lubes, the taste of come, fellatio games, role-play, bondage, pairing anal play with fellatio, and much more.

So, sit back, relax, and enjoy this information-packed, sexy read. There are many fun tricks and techniques to try, adorable illustrations by Molly Kiely, and steamy, explicit short stories by Alison Tyler to get you hot and bothered. May you enjoy putting this book into practice as much as I have enjoyed doing the research.

Violet Blue
Berkeley, CA
August 2002

More Than a Mouthful

Fellatio is a versatile and wonderful erotic art that you can use in any type of sex play with your male (or strap-on-wearing) partner. You can take him in your mouth during foreplay, in between your favorite sex positions, or when switching erotic activities; swap oral favors in a 69; or save fellatio for your last course, dessert. It can be a teasing taste of what's to come later, a clandestine moment, a tit-for-tat trade, or the entire delicious menu. Oral sex can add intimacy to your relationships, and if you don't already include it in your repertoire, going down on him can bring you both closer together. However you choose to incorporate it, whatever you like to call it—*fellatio, blow job, hummer, giving head*—the only limitations on how you can use it to enhance your lovemaking are in your mind. The possibilities are endless.

My husband and I like to pretend I'm a prostitute when I go down on him. It feels dirty and bad, and I like it.

This book is a terrific starting point for people who have never gone down on a man before. In these pages you'll find all the accurate sex information you need to make your first experience safe, pleasurable, and successful. Or if you're a seasoned pro, you will find plenty of new ideas to try with your favorite fellatio partner. Learning about his sexual anatomy from a pleasure perspective will give you a road map to guide your oral encounters, and you'll see how his penis, testicles, and anus like to be touched. You'll also learn about the stages of the male arousal cycle and what happens when men get turned on and when they orgasm—and how to read their body language throughout the process. The essential components of fellatio to orgasm are covered in detail, and you'll learn how to use your mouth and hands in many delightful combinations. In addition, you will learn how to get off while you go down, get comfortable with deep throating, and layer oodles of tricks and techniques onto your own personal style of giving head.

So Nice to Get, So Nice to Give

The moment she started sucking, it was incredible. I still don't know why it was so excellent. Part of it was because I was in love with her, and because I had been craving that she suck my cock. But there was a purely physical, sensual aspect to it, which was perfect—beyond anything I had experienced.

Why do men enjoy getting head? A soft pair of lips kissing; a warm and wet tongue caressing; a whole hot mouth wrapped around the center of his pleasure—this, for many men, is heaven on earth. Our mouths convey a sensation unlike any other and can easily stimulate a

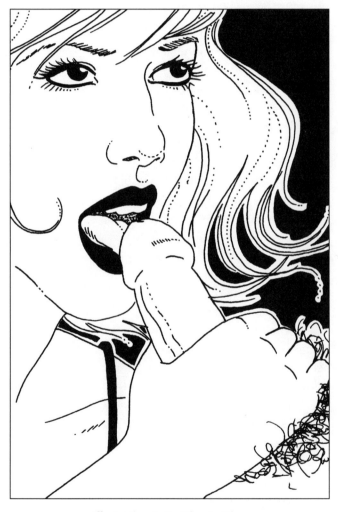

Illustration 1. So Nice to Give

man to the point of no return. Hands, sex toys, vaginas, breasts, and butts all have their rightful places in the world of sex play, but fellatio combines these elements seamlessly for focused, powerful orgasms that include just as powerful visual stimulation for the recipient.

I love watching girls giving head.

When you go down on a guy, he gets much more than your velvety mouth and a pair of luscious lips wrapped around him. Men love the physical sensations that go along with fellatio, but some even get off on the peripherals—the visual and mental stimulation—more than the sensations. When a lover is between a man's legs, he has a clear view of all the action, from beginning to end. He sees and feels everything you do. And because most everyone likes some form of visual stimulation, head can be one of the ultimate sex shows—starring him and you. Some men enjoy seeing it as a form of devotion in which they are being lovingly worshiped, adored, made love to. Others might get off on the feeling of power, relishing the notion of being "serviced" or even "taking" the pleasure you offer.

Many men who like oral sex see it simply as that: oral sex, nothing more than a wonderful variation on the menu of sex acts from which you both may choose. It feels good, it feels divine, it's another fun thing to do with a lover. Another man may think it's very special and intimate to have a lover who genuinely wants to make him feel good by going down on him. In this case, oral sex is a deliberately shared act that connects body and heart.

Oral sex with a man can happen anywhere. That's part of the pleasure. And time and place adds to his experience. In the office after hours, it's naughty, sexy, on the sly. A bedroom can make it more comfortable and private, allowing a broader range of sex play—fellatio as a part of sex that can include one or many different acts in an evening. There are more devious places, such as bathroom stalls and other semipublic settings, where the sheer wickedness of fellatio combined with the risk of being discovered add to the charge of the experience.

Getting Head: Check Your Assumptions at the Door

There's a particular emotional sense of being fully accepted that I feel when a woman gives me head that adds to my pleasure. You'd think that's what intercourse is for, but to tell you the truth, I actually experience that sense of total acceptance more strongly when I receive oral sex.

For most men, the thought of an enthusiastic pair of lips wrapping around their penis triggers a response similar to that of a popsicle being similarly sucked—they melt. Getting head is often one of his favorite things; there is really nothing that can duplicate the feeling of a mouth and tongue, supply the arousing visual stimulation, or communicate the acceptance found within the act of his lover kissing his most intimate physical place, his genitals. When you fellate your lover, you make him feel incredibly good physically, stimulate his fantasies (or participate in the creation of new ones for him to revisit later), and make love to him in a direct way, face-to-cock—a way that says "I want you" loud and clear.

It's a commonly accepted cultural idea that head—and all the wonderful things associated with getting it—is what every man wants. Also wrapped in society's onionlike layers of assumptions surrounding fellatio are two oversimplified stereotypes about men and sex: that men always want it, because penises are like machines and can just plug in anywhere anytime, and that men want head because it's like an instant service, akin to dropping off the laundry. Not to say that for some men these perspectives aren't true—they may be true for a few men most of the time, and other men might feel this way only occasionally, while others seldom, if ever. But in reality, these assumptions and stereotypes about fellatio only serve to distance us from our lovers. A cock is not a lightbulb. Its owner might even have concerns about getting a blow job.

Men can feel stress about receiving oral sex. Having someone look at, watch the reactions of, smell, and taste your genitals is an intense experience for anyone—especially in our world of constant comparisons. He might be worried about his performance, size, or shape, or whether he's responding appropriately to your touch. He might also be contending with sexual shame, which can cloud his ability to relax, let go, and enjoy what you're doing. These anxieties are not limited to men—we all have issues regarding sexual comparisons and shame, which come from the culture we've grown up in. But oral sex in particular can bring these issues into sharp focus. If you feel as though your partner might have questions or anxieties about receiving fellatio, encourage him to read chapter 3, "For Him," in which I cover men's oral sex anxieties in detail.

Giving Head: Eye of the Beholder

Nothing makes me wet like when I feel him get extra hard in my mouth and then the spasms begin... I love to feel him come, really feel it come out of him, and have it shoot onto the back of my tongue and in my throat.

Going down on a man is one of life's singular pleasures. Nothing compares to having the absolute focus
of your lover's heat, intensity, lust, and desire right in
front of you, and in your mouth. You hold his enjoyment and his orgasm within the confines of your body.
Make it a long, loving tribute, a gentle massage, a prolonged seduction, or a quick and dirty episode that you
both share—it can be anything you like. Giving our
lovers pleasure gives us pleasure, too. For some who like
to give, it's more a pleasure of the heart, mind, or soul;
for others, it's a direct pathway to their own arousal; or
it can be both.

In a very general sense, there are two ways in which
a blow job can be performed. There is *fellatio,* the tech-
nical term used to describe the act of a person going up
and down on the penis; and there is *irrumation,* in which
the giver stays stationary and the man receiving the blow
job provides the in-and-out motion with his thrusting.
However, *fellatio* is the colloquial blanket term for all
things blow job, and that's how I'll be using the word
throughout this book.

The idea of performing fellatio makes some people
anxious, uncomfortable, even afraid. If you're one of
those people, then you may dislike feeling that oral sex
is purely for the enjoyment of the person on the receiving side. You may not consider fellatio to be a sexually
mutual act—especially if your perception of oral sex in
general is negative.

Our culture perpetuates the image of the sexually
receptive partner as being submissive; the very act of
receipt is often thought of as a brand of humiliation and
shame. It's tough enough to shrug this notion off of how
we view penetrative sex (vaginal and anal), but when
it comes to fellatio, cultural perceptions everywhere

suggest that anyone willing to put a guy's penis in his or her mouth is dirty and disposable, and deserves no respect. However, these myths exist only in the eye of the beholder; any sex act between two people is what you make it.

Mixed into the myth of the soiled cocksucker is the idea that fellatio is done solely for the pleasure of the person getting the blow job. For as many people who believe this, there are probably twice as many who get wet or stiff from going down on a guy. The mouth is an erogenous zone that triggers erotic responses, and for many people simply the act of taking him in their mouth (or just the idea of it) can trigger powerful arousal or even orgasm.

If you still feel uncomfortable about fellatio, indulge me for a moment and try on a new idea, just to see how it feels: the flip side. Many people view taking a man's erect penis into their mouth as an act of unrivaled intimacy and sharing. For some people, being up close to his most private areas, face-to-face with his pleasure, able to kiss and adore him in the most immediate way, is a closeness that can't be found in other sex acts. Many people find oral sex to be more intimate than intercourse. That he feels comfortable with your face in close contact with his genitals is an erotically charged gift of unrivaled trust. Plus, the fact that you can see his desire for you, and he can see yours for him, right there, makes it a delicious moment of sharing.

> *The connection I feel with my partner while getting head is amazing. There's nothing more beautiful—it's like the hottest, sexiest thing I can be engaged in, and the more I know she's enjoying it, the hotter it is.*

You've probably heard this phrase, or something similar: "Who do I have to blow to get a cup of coffee around here?" It's a stereotypical perception in our culture to regard blow jobs as a commodity, effectively removing the "sex" from the act. But it's a sexual act, and quite an intense one for the giver and the receiver. It's confusing to reconcile these two views, and the end result is often a perception of giving head as a sex act that reduces the giver's status. When people joke about giving head for coffee, then what's the worth of the person going down? It's this way of looking at fellatio that makes it easy to think of giving blow jobs—and sex in general—as degrading.

If you're reluctant to try fellatio, or you feel bad when you do it, examine where these feelings are coming from. Sexual shame is a learned behavior, and if we want to, we can unlearn negative attitudes about sex. Are you worried that he'll have less respect for you if you give him head? Worried that you'll respect yourself less? Ask yourself why you feel this way about your lover, yourself, and fellatio. If he's the type of person who treats you negatively after fellatio, then he's certainly going to treat you negatively in all other aspects of intimate contact, and you should ask yourself some tough questions about your relationship.

If your feelings are directed inward, or if you have an imaginary gallery of judges in your head, ask yourself how realistic you're being about your feelings and where they stem from. Are you being too hard on yourself? Do you really want to be with this person? What do you think is going to change after you go down on a man? Who taught you to feel this way about fellatio, and does it make sense to you? These questions are not easy to answer. But if you are ashamed about a sex act that you'd like to try, you'll feel better and enjoy your-self more if you understand why you're feeling the way you are.

If you're working on your level of comfort with fel-latio, you can put a few things into practice to help you along. Reading this book and finding concrete answers to your questions is a great place to start. There are exer-cises in these pages that you'll want to try, such as practicing on a dildo so you can get used to fellatio's physical sensations. Talking to your lover is another way to establish comfort, and you can voice concerns you might have, such as worries about gagging, or let him know if you don't want him to come in your mouth or put his hands on your head. You can also try situations or positions that will address your concerns: giving a blow job in the shower will ensure cleanliness, having him lie flat on his back will give you the most control. Whether or not he ejaculates in your mouth is up to you, and you can address this in different ways. Should you decide that you'd rather he didn't, you can discuss a signal he can give you before he's going to come (for instance, giving you a tap on the shoulder), and you can have him come elsewhere. Techniques for this are pre-sented in chapter 7, "Giving Head."

> She has long, deep red hair that's slightly wavy and very thick. Fantastic to run my fingers through during sex and especially during a blow job.

> I hate even thinking about having a guy hold my head when I suck him. I tried it once and it felt like I was going to suffocate!

High on the list of givers' concerns about fellatio is the notion of control: giving head can sometimes make you feel vulnerable, as if the person you're performing the act on has more power than you. In this scenario the fear is of being pushed too far, beyond your own boundaries, for someone else's sexual satisfaction. You might be afraid that he's going to thrust uncontrollably into your mouth, or grab your head and hold you down. Be up front with him about where you stand with having your head touched before his pants are unzipped. If you don't get this chance, but decide to go down anyway, decide that if he touches your head you're just going to stop what you're doing, move his hands to his own body, then proceed. He should get the message. For techniques and positions that can help you counter the movements of a man who thrusts uncontrollably, see chapter 8, "Any Way You Want It."

> *When I had less experience with blow jobs I worried about whether he was clean or not. I was always worried that he'd smell like pee or something, and it really freaked me out. Now I've done it several times, and it's never as gross as I thought it might be.*

Perhaps you're not as worried about whether it's a dirty thing to do as you are about whether he's the dirty one—literally. Growing up, we're all taught that sex organs are dirty, and it's hard to shake this view as we become adults. Because we tend to see genitals as unclean, the idea of putting a penis in your mouth may make you think twice. If you find yourself feeling this way, get the facts on male anatomy and physiology in chapter 2, "The Anatomy of a Man's Pleasure," before you go any further. If you're with a new partner and are worried about sexually transmitted diseases, read about what fellatio can put you at risk for in chapter 4, "Know the Hard Facts: Health Considerations." But if you're already aware of the facts and still feel reluctant, try catching him after he takes a shower, or try taking a seductive bath together before fellatio; this way you'll know he's squeaky clean.

> *I was pretty scared the first time I went down on a guy, but it turned out fine. We were in the bathtub, and when he came I hardly noticed because everything was already wet.*

If you have concerns about safer sex, cleanliness, or other health issues, your concerns are covered in later chapters. Get the facts about what you need to know, and then you can make an informed decision based on your own comfort level. He may have a few concerns of his own, especially if he's never tried it before (or tried it with you), so feel free to point him to chapters of this book to allay fears, dispel myths, or simply answer any questions he might have.

Talk About It

If you're chomping on the bit to give your lover some oral sex that will feel genuinely pleasurable, you want to go down and he's reluctant to let you, or you want to change something about fellatio in your sex life, then talking about it will give you a starting point. Not every man in the world has had a blow job, so it's possible that you're reading this book wanting to give or get head for the first time. Also, some men who have received fellatio have not enjoyed it, and telling your partner what you like or dislike, or asking him what stimulation he enjoys, can seem daunting. It's also possible that you're reading this from the perspective of wanting to give or receive strap-on fellatio, but need a way to introduce the act to your existing partnership.

Talking to your partner about sex can feel stressful. In fact, even thinking about talking about sex is stressful sometimes! If you've never brought up the subject of sex with your partner, don't worry. Telling your partner that you want something in your sex life to change is scary if you have a routine. Opening yourself up and asking for something you want sexually takes courage, strategy, and a little forethought about why your partner might be reluctant. Just keep in mind that in all matters of sex, it will only happen if someone is brave enough to say, "I want to…"

If you're planning to introduce a new erotic behavior, such as fellatio or strap-on cocksucking, or want to change the way you have oral sex together, you're probably wondering how your partner will react. When you don't normally talk about sex in your relationship and one of you suddenly starts to, it can seem upsetting at first. Your lover may wonder if you've had sexual secrets all along. But it's very likely that your opening up the can of worms will give them the opportunity to tell you what's on their mind about sex, too.

Before you begin, think about how you might bring up the subject in a way that would feel safe for you: Would you feel more comfortable renting a mainstream movie with an oral sex scene in it, and commenting on the scene (some possibilities are *Two Guys and a Girl, Pretty Woman, Boogie Nights,* or *Body of Evidence*)? Or do you think you'd feel okay asking your sweetie what he thinks of fellatio while you're entwined in an intimate cuddle? Try giving him a collection of erotic stories as a gift, or read aloud a story that contains a fellatio scene that's to your liking (see the book recommendations in chapter 12, "Independent Study"). Another technique you can try is telling him you want to confess a fantasy—a sexual fantasy—and that he isn't to reply right away. Tell him that you can have a conversation about it later; this gives both parties time to feel safe about the exchange.

Consider ways in which you can encourage your partner to hear you out, and ask them to suspend judgment until you can explain why this is important, and how good this new sexual behavior is going to make you feel—and be sure to reassure them that you find them incredibly sexy. Whether you're reading this from the perspective of wanting to give or receive head, the most important thing to think through beforehand is how you are going to make your partner feel safe when talking about it. Rehearse what you'd like to say in your head before you actually have the conversation. Think through possible scenarios, and think about how they might react, so you are prepared to flow with whichever route the discussion might take.

The idea of having your face between their legs might make some men anxious. Before you open the discussion, you'll want to read up on the fears and issues that men face in chapter 3, "For Him." If you can get a handle on what might be bothering him before you open the discussion, you can listen more sympathetically, knowing a little bit about what could be on his mind.

When Your Lover Is Reluctant

When you want to give your sweetie sexual pleasure and he's reluctant, nonresponsive, or seems unsure, it can be a little deflating—and confusing. Understanding why he is hesitant or where this hesitation might be coming from is important if you want to reverse any negative sexual messages he might be dealing with. There are a number of reasons why your lover might be hesitant, and sexual shame is a biggie. No matter how you were raised, you most certainly learned on one level or another that sex is "bad," were made to feel that you should have a "perfect" body, and were taught that genitals are "icky." Through advertising, pop culture, and conservative religious and social mores, our culture repeats to us over and over that we should be ashamed of our bodies, our sexual selves, afraid of expressing natural, healthy sexuality.

Many people consider oral sex to be more intimate than intercourse. Some men might find that having you up close and personal with their penis magnifies worries, concerns, and insecurities. He might worry about how he looks, how he compares, how he might taste or smell, or if he will have a trustworthy erection. Some guys feel unsettled by the intimacy of being in your mouth and your ability to watch his reactions; even the sheer closeness of the act might make them nervous. Some men just don't like their bodies and won't want you to get a close look. These are all very good reasons why he might be apprehensive about having you go down on him. Be sensitive, and ask questions gently in hopes of creating a space in which your partner will feel safe to open up about his hesitancy. Trust takes time to build, even in long-term relationships, but he may eventually come to love his genitals, sex, and intimacy as much as you do.

If he's partially open to the idea but still hesitant, try engaging in foreplay (such as male genital massage; for more on this see chapter 6, "Before You Go Down") up to his threshold of comfort, and then switch to a sexual activity that's comfortable for both of you. Next time you try, go up to that point and a little past it, slowly easing up to fellatio. If his anxiety stems from issues with cleanliness, taste, or smell, you can romantically shower or bathe together beforehand. If it seems appropriate and you're both turned on, initiate oral sex in the shower. If he's uncomfortable with his genitals being in your mouth, it's a good idea to keep a wet washcloth at your bedside, because he probably won't want to be kissed after getting head. If you know he's uncomfortable about body size or how his body looks in general, plan your seduction by romantic candlelight or use lowered ambient light—or the two of you can stay partially clothed during sex.

A concern among some men is that they'll lose their erection during fellatio, which is the worst possible moment—when he knows you're trying to give him pleasure, and you're watching him. Let him know that you understand the rising and falling of the male pleasure cycle, and just enjoy having him in your mouth. Many men really enjoy having their soft penis lovingly kissed, sucked, and cradled in a warm mouth, so you can continue to fellate him if he becomes soft. It feels great to him—having an erection isn't required to have hot sex. Penises don't stop receiving pleasure when they're not hard, and neither do their owners! Tell him that you don't care if he's hard during your pleasure play, as long as he's involved. Or tell him you're orally fixated, and he's helping you quit smoking! But seriously, this issue can nag even the most sexually confident man, and it's your responsibility to tell him that your goal is simply shared pleasure. Let him know that if he gets hard and orgasms, that's great, and if not, it's just as great—you're making love to the man, not the body part. Do what you can to ease any pressure he may be feeling about "getting it up," and he'll be able to enjoy what you're doing for his own sake. Talk to him about this: great lovers ask questions, lousy lovers don't.

Trying New Things

If you want to perform fellatio and never have before, you're going to be adding a new dimension to your sexuality. If you're in a relationship and are interested in trying it, you're adding a new sexual behavior to your routine. Or fellatio may already be part of your lovemaking, but one of you wants it to change. Adding new sex practices or tailoring existing ones to heighten the experience of sex can be a lot of fun—or it can be a nerve-wracking experience.

The important thing to consider when adding any new sexual technique to your repertoire is where your goals lie. Are you interested in increasing intimacy, or do you just want to get off? Is your goal to establish trust, or to have an evening of arousing, teasing sexual play? Is it orgasm, foreplay, affection, or fun you're after? Regardless, you'll want to make your main goal to have fun, be close, and deeply lust after your lover. If you're hot for what you're doing to him, he'll be able to tell, no matter what oral technique you're trying to perfect. And if he's feeling your heat for what you both are doing, then you've got yourself a peak erotic experience in the making.

2

The Anatomy of a Man's Pleasure

Is seems so simple, doesn't it? What guys like, that is. To the casual observer, male genital physiology is but one step away from "tab A into slot B." But that's a misconception—in fact, there's a lot more going on down there than meets the eye. When we think of pleasing our male partners, we think it's easy to do. Sometimes that's true, but when you discover just how much pleasure he's capable of receiving, you'll want to leave the easy stuff to the amateurs.

Appearance and Pleasure Physiology

Men's genitals are as unique as a face or a fingerprint. But though there are infinite variations, what you will generally encounter when you unzip his fly is a penis (circumcised or not), a scrotal sack containing two testicles, and pubic hair that usually covers the mound over the pubic bone, the base of the penis, the testicles, and the perineum (from the base of the balls to the anus). The skin on the pubic mound, the perineum, and the anus is similar in texture to the skin on the rest of his

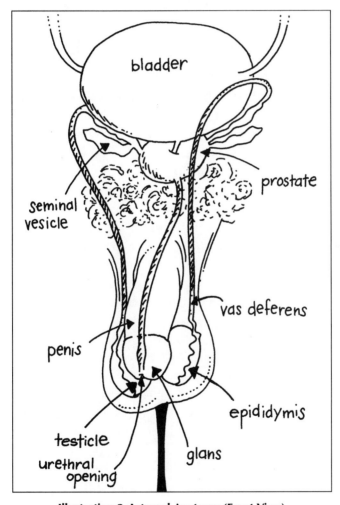

Illustration 2. Internal Anatomy (Front View)

body, but usually a different shade. It deepens and changes in color as it reaches the base of the penis and the scrotum. The darker skin is softer and thinner than the skin on the rest of his body.

We'll begin with the front and work our way back. Penises come in a variety of shapes and sizes. The range of sensation is also different for each man and depends on various factors—so rule number one is that you can't predict anything based on the way a penis looks. The base of the penis sprouts from the pubic mound, which is usually covered with hair—it can be thick as a forest, or thin and barely there. The skin covering the pubic bone (or pubic mound) is generally fleshier than any of the skin surrounding it, and the mound is where the skin begins to deepen in color as it meets the base of the penis. The shaft of the penis begins just below the pubic bone and continues internally almost all the way to the anus.

Nature loves variety, and men's penises are no exception. Penises come in more shapes, sizes, and variations than words can communicate—though there certainly has been a lot written about them. The skin covering a man's penis is almost always darker in tone than the skin everywhere else (though sometimes it's lighter), and it's more smooth in texture. Colors can range from the lightest pink to the deepest chocolate and anywhere in between. The color at the tip, also called the *head,* or *glans,* will generally differ from the rest of the penis, especially his circumcision scar (if he has one), and penises are seldom the same color all over. They also vary greatly in size, both in flaccid (soft) and erect (hard) states. The size of a man's soft penis is not a reliable gauge of his erect state—again, you can't tell just by looking. Shapes are yet another variable: he can be thick at the base and slender at the tip, wide from top to bottom, with a wide head but slender in girth, or any number of combinations, each of which is perfectly normal. The color, size, and shape of a man's penis has nothing to do with how he responds to stimulation—or what type of lover he is.

The penis is essentially a long shaft, or tube, that ends at the tip with the urethral opening, where urine and ejaculate (sperm or "come") leave the body. Inside the penis, the urethra continues as a long tube through the center of two other larger tubes of spongy erectile tissue, whose proper names are *corpus cavernosum* and *corpus spongiosum*. When arousal triggers an erection, these tissues fill with blood, hardening the shaft and head of his penis. However, an erection does not always indicate whether a man is aroused; he can be perfectly, happily aroused and remain unerect.

At the tip is where you'll find the head, or glans. The head has the largest concentration of nerve endings in the penis, and it can be very responsive to stimulation—sometimes extremely sensitive to touch (especially after orgasm). Always ask your partner what level of stimulation works for him at any given time with the head of his cock, because his preference levels will change throughout the pleasure cycle. The head is often bulbous—anywhere from slightly to quite pronounced. If he's uncircumcised, in its soft state the head will be covered in a thin jacket of skin called a *foreskin*. As his penis becomes aroused, the glans will harden and emerge. In North America, most infant boys are circumcised, a process in which the foreskin is removed after the bundle of joy is delivered.

Beneath the head of his cock is usually the most sensitive part, which some men claim is their "sweet spot," the spot they really enjoy having touched when they're aroused. This spot can range in location from just at the urethral opening to farther down the underside of the shaft, where the circumcision scar lies. On an uncircumcised man, this spot runs along the same area, beneath the tip of the cockhead, from the urethral opening (underside) to approximately where the inner skin of the foreskin's hood meets the outer skin of the penis.

Cut or Uncut?

Most American men have circumcised penises, meaning that the foreskins were removed from their penises shortly after they were born. The foreskin, which they no longer have, is a thin jacket of skin that covers the head tightly, like a wetsuit, with an opening that allows urine to leave the body. When an uncircumcised man is aroused, his cock stiffens and the head swells, emerging from under the hood of the foreskin, which often—but not always—retracts.

On an "uncut" penis, the outer surface of the foreskin consists of skin similar to that on the rest of the penis. Inside the foreskin is an inner layer of very sensitive, moist mucosal tissue, similar to the skin of the inner labia in women. Connecting the foreskin to the penis is the *frenulum,* which is where the foreskin is cut away during circumcision. When aroused and stroked by a hand, a mouth, or anything else pleasurable, the foreskin is mostly retracted but slides up and down pleasurably on his frenulum, a sensation many men consider exquisite.

Some people are nervous about going down on uncircumcised men. Most of this anxiety comes from not understanding what's different about having a foreskin—if you have not seen an uncut penis before, it

might look different from most others you have encoun-
tered and even appear to respond differently. If your
partner is uncircumcised and you have concerns about
how to stimulate him, ask. He's probably been asked
before; even if he has not, he would probably love
the chance to tell a lover who cares enough to ask
exactly how he likes to be touched. Another concern
people might have when first encountering a foreskin is
cleanliness—how do guys get it clean in there? Most
uncircumcised men learned at an early age how to pull
back the skin in the shower and apply soap and water.
But if you're really worried, then suggest a shower
together, and you can delight him with your inquisitive
and arousing washing techniques.

The Testicles

Underneath the penis is where we find the scrotal sack,
containing the testicles (or testicle—not all men have
a pair). These are the "balls." Their wrinkly, fleshy container, the *scrotum* (or scrotal sack), hangs attached at
the base of his penis and can be the same color as the
penis or darker in tone. With rare exceptions, the testicles are usually covered with a lighter covering of hair
than the pubic bone, yet they can sometimes be just as
furry. Most men's testicles hang unevenly; one is usually
lower than the other. According to a 1996 *Men's Health*
survey of over 2000 readers, in 85 percent of men the
left testicle is the lower one.

The scrotum is a container of loose, thin skin that
holds the testicles inside. Its unusual characteristic is the
cremaster muscle, which causes the testicles to wrinkle
here and there and to go up and down as they contract
and relax. It's really a heat regulator: when it's chilly, the
muscle will pull the scrotum up and the testicles close to

the body, and when the temperature rises, it relaxes and lets them hang. Before he's about to ejaculate, the muscle retracts, pulling the testicles close to the base of the penis.

Inside the scrotal sack lie one, two, or sometimes three testicles—though you will most often find two. Men can have one, two, or more testicles from the time they are born, or they might later have one (or more) removed for medical reasons, such as cancer. These small, egg-shaped spheres feel uneven and bumpy in texture when you touch them through the skin, but that's because they're tightly wound masses that consist of tubes—similar to a rubber-band ball. Between the tubes are cells that produce that celebrity hormone testosterone, and the tubes themselves are where sperm are born and bred. The sperm travel from the tubes through a lumpy mass at the back of the testicle that's actually one long coiled-up tube, and into the fast freeway of the *vas deferens*. Destination: urethra.

A man's testicles are very sensitive to the touch, but many men enjoy having them caressed, lightly massaged, or even gently tugged or pulled during foreplay and arousal. Most men will not enjoy having them slapped, spanked, or even sucked—but there are exceptions, and this type of pleasure play should be expressly discussed in advance. Generally, you should treat them like a pair of delicate eggs.

Behind the testicles and between the thighs is a flat stretch of skin that's also covered with hair and often the same color as the penis—this is his *perineum*. Beneath the skin of the perineum is where the root, or bulb, of the penis lies, and when he gets an erection you can feel this area harden, too. Stroke or rub this area during other sexual stimulation, and you will probably get a positive response.

The Anus and Prostate

The prostate gland is the starlet gland of the male body. It is at once villain and vixen: the seat of the most-diagnosed cancer in men, and the possible promise of pleasure from beyond the stars. Rebuked, reviled,

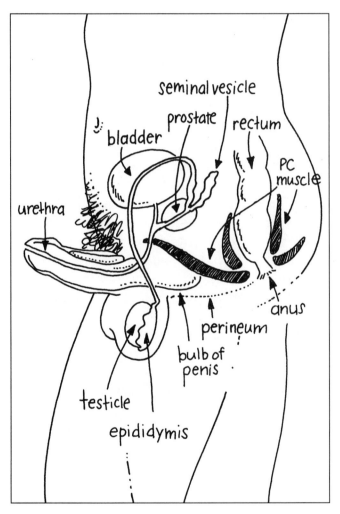

Illustration 3. Internal Anatomy (Side View)

redeemed, and romanced, this little gland manages to make headlines when viewed from any angle. Sometimes the attention is conflicted: the gland makes prostatic fluid for carrying virile semen, making the man "a man"; it also makes orgasm outrageously powerful but requires access through anal penetration, questioning some people's definition of "a man."

Not all men enjoy anal stimulation—whether it's gentle touching on the outside, rimming, or penetration and prostate stimulation—but many men find that it adds a new dimension to sex play. One of the reasons that men like anal play is because massaging the prostate gland feels incredibly pleasurable and can make orgasm very powerful, but they might also like it because the anus and anal opening is rich with nerve endings that feel good to the touch, or for various psychological reasons. He may like that it's a big taboo, that it's a "dirty" thing to do; maybe no one touches him there and it means a lot to have you care about his pleasure; or it may be part of a dominant/submissive fantasy scenario in which he "makes" you do it, or you "make" him submit to it. One thing is certain—the men who like anal stimulation during fellatio like it a lot, and for many of these men, prostate stimulation can turn a good blow job into an unforgettable experience.

The perineum stretches from the base of the testicles to the anus, where it is no longer perineum and definitely ass. It has some hair, either a light, downy covering, or a thick, coarse carpet—it's different on every man. All humans have hair around their anus, whatever your gender; if you don't, then you either shave it or are too young to be reading this. Between his cheeks, you'll see the anal opening, a pucker that will differ in color from the skin on the rest of the body. In fact, it's common for the thin skin surrounding the pucker to be lighter or darker in color between the cheeks.

The prostate gland is within the front wall of the anal opening, usually around 1 to 3 inches inside and forward (toward the front of the body or belly button). Its location inside the wall is just behind the bulb of the penis, beneath the bladder, surrounding the urethra in a ring. Because the prostate is anchored at the internal base of the penis, when a man thrusts hard with an erect penis he transmits highly pleasurable sensations to the prostate. It's a little larger than a quarter in size, though it is heart-shaped and is usually described as being the size of a small walnut.

Surprisingly little is known about the prostate gland. It produces prostatic fluid (the whitish liquid that carries sperm during ejaculation), it grows as a man ages (sometimes dangerously), and it can feel really, really good when sexually stimulated. It's clear that it plays an important role in the male pleasure cycle, and it has become touted as the male G-spot. When a man reaches the point of orgasmic "no return" (ejaculatory inevitability), the prostate gland joins the seminal vesicles and other ducts in pleasant-feeling spasms and rhythmic contractions to create ejaculate—and this is before the contractions of orgasm. If you are stimulating a man's prostate prior to and during ejaculation, you can often feel the gland swell to hardness, then contract before his orgasm.

To feel the prostate, insert a well-lubricated finger inside his anal opening and stroke toward the front of his body, in a "come-hither" motion. It may be too soft to feel easily in its unaroused state; in fact, you may not be able to feel it at all until he becomes aroused, when it swells and hardens. Similarly to the G-spot in women, the prostate may trigger the feeling of needing to urinate when stroked. For men who aren't ready for penetration, you can stimulate the prostate indirectly by massaging the perineum in firm circles with the flat of your thumb. Some men like perineum massage only when they're aroused, and some don't like it at all—when in doubt, ask. For prostate stimulation tips and techniques for fellatio, read chapter 10, "More Techniques."

His Sexual Response Cycle

When a man becomes aroused, his senses go into overdrive. The everyday becomes the superreal; his sense of smell is heightened, colors are brighter, his skin becomes more sensitive and responds readily to touch. Whatever was sexy to him before he got turned on is even more sexy, and his focus is hormonally sharpened on just one thing: more pleasure. Meanwhile, his internal and external sexual anatomy are responding—big time. Many different muscles involuntarily tense, resulting in contractions of facial and abdominal muscles. His breathing becomes heavier, his core body temperature rises, his heart rate increases, his nipples may become erect, and some men get a sex flush across their chest, neck, face, and stomach. And if his penis begins to become erect, the head darkens in color and his testicles swell and move close to his body.

Arousal triggers physical reactions, but it doesn't necessarily have to come from a physical source. Physiological arousal can come from either of two sources or, more likely, a combination of the two—mentally, from his brain, or physically, from his body's response to stimulation. These two factors need each other to create physiological arousal, though they can operate at varying levels: in a given instance, fantasy may be fueling the fires more than touch, or vice-versa. The mind and body work in tandem to make a man hot under the collar and hard under the Calvins—you can have one without the other and still be aroused, but then, well, you have one and not the other. These two factors (in whatever proportion) trigger neural responses along nerve pathways that widen the arteries leading to the penis and other erectile tissue. Blood begins to flow into his penis and its underground erectile tissue, and his penis and perineum begin to harden. The prostate starts to grow firm to the touch.

Blood flows into the main tubes of the penis, creating rigidity as the flow of blood expands the erectile tissue, trapping the blood in his penis, creating and sustaining the erection until the nerve messages stop, or he ejaculates. (The nerve pathways for erection and ejaculation are different, which is why a man can ejaculate without erection and vice-versa.) The blood flowing to his genitals is also being trapped inside in the bulb and root of his penis, contributing to a firmer perineum.

To make an erection, the blood swells the tissue inside until it strains against the sheath of skin covering the penis. Lo, it is risen. The head also swells, and in uncircumcised men this swelling pushes the glans forward out of the opening in the foreskin. Erections come in many flavors—soft, semisoft, hard, rock-hard—and can fill out the shape of the penis differently depending on the man. When erect, he may be straight as a board, curve up, down, left, or right, or be firmer at one end than the other. As his pleasure cycle moves up and down the peaks and valleys of arousal, so will his erection grow soft and firm again. In prolonged sexual encounters, it's not uncommon for erections to come and go as the lovemaking session progresses, and this normal cycling has nothing to do with his actual arousal or desire.

At the urethral opening, during arousal some men get wet with what's commonly called *pre-come*. This clear fluid usually appears when he's really turned on, and while some men have only a little, others can be quite juicy. It also changes in amount from one experience to another; he might be really wet sometimes, while other times he's not wet at all. Pre-come is a combination of the fluid forced from the walls of the urethra and ejaculatory fluids produced in the prostatic urethra (where the fluids mix with semen before ejaculation). Pre-come contains semen, and it can contain viruses if your partner has one, so it's important to treat it just as you would ejaculate—with all the necessary safer-sex precautions. (For information on safer sex, see chapter 4, "Know the Hard Facts: Health Considerations.")

As his arousal heightens, all the muscles and ligaments in the genital region begin to tighten, creating an exquisite tension. The prostate gland is swollen with fluid, waiting for the signal to begin its contractions. The figure eight of muscles that surround the penile system and ring the anus become tense, creating more pleasure and making his entire lower body part of the pleasure process.

> *I hold my boyfriend's balls while I suck him off. He likes it, and as they get tighter I can tell he's about to come.*

Muscle tension builds to a pinnacle as he reaches the point of no return. His glans is very sensitive to stimulation, and both penis and shaft become very hard, as does the prostate. The testicles pull up very close to his body, contributing a delicious pressure. His breathing is labored, his blood pressure is up, and the skin all over his body is electric and extremely sensitive. His whole body is flooded with potent sexual chemicals, coloring his vision with nothing but the demands of getting more of whatever is pushing him onward. Before the peak, the prostate gland shudders and releases the prostatic fluid to mix with semen and other juices—this is "orgasmic inevitability," the point when a man knows he is about to come, and nothing on earth can stop it. Then the short, rhythmic muscular contractions of orgasm begin, not just in the penis but also throughout the entire genital region (including the sphincter muscle), and he orgasms, usually with ejaculation. This is the moment of pure pleasure. And with a little experimentation, men can orgasm multiple times and in many ways.

Ejaculation

During the orgasmic phase of sexual response, when a man feels orgasmic inevitability, the fluids that comprise ejaculatory fluid are being pushed into the prostatic urethra. This makes him feel like he's about to come. When the involuntary muscular contractions of orgasm begin, the muscles of his penis and urethra squeeze the opening to his bladder completely closed, and the seminal fluid (now mixed with sperm) shoots out of his penis. Ejaculation is usually accompanied by the rhythmic contractions of the pelvic muscles, though it's possible to ejaculate without orgasm, and it's also possible for him to orgasm without ejaculation.

Most men ejaculate when they orgasm, but not all do, and not all men ejaculate every time. A man may not ejaculate due to frequent ejaculation, because of health issues such as retrograde ejaculation, or because he has learned how to orgasm without ejaculating using a technique for male multiple orgasms. If he has been ejaculating frequently or is having several orgasms in one session of sex, the amount of fluid he expels will decrease, sometimes until it seems like nothing is coming out. Retrograde ejaculation is when the opening, or valve, between the bladder and the urethra doesn't close during the muscular contractions of orgasm. When this happens, ejaculatory fluid is sent into the bladder. Retrograde ejaculation generally occurs in men who have spinal cord injuries or have had prostate or bladder surgery. This should not interfere with the pleasure of orgasm, but if there is pain or discomfort, he should see a doctor.

The Multi-Orgasmic Man, by Douglas Abrams Arava and Mantak Chia, has revolutionized the way Western men control their orgasms. The book teaches men techniques that employ pressure points, controlled breathing, and muscular control to change the way they orgasm. Orgasms can be strengthened, lengthened, and multiplied; it's also possible for men to learn how to orgasm without ejaculation. With a little practice, a man can experience the pleasure of full-body orgasms, along with all the accompanying muscular contractions, without expelling the usual mass of ejaculatory fluid. Some men may have come across their own techniques for this through experimentation. Keep in mind that this is by no means a substitute for safer-sex practices and should never be considered a reliable form of birth control.

Men who ejaculate expel different amounts, but it's usually around 1 to 2 teaspoons. The volume can change depending on frequency (whether he's come recently, or not in a long time), stress, or other factors. Come is comprised of plasma, fluid from the prostate and seminal vesicles, around 90 million sperm, and other fluids that contain fructose, protein, citric acid, alkalines, and other nutrients that keep sperm intact. It can also contain HIV and sexually transmitted diseases, if he's infected. Come is usually whitish in color, but the color can also be varying degrees of clear, white, or yellow. The texture is that of a slightly thick liquidy substance, somewhere between egg whites and hair conditioner, though some men might have very thick come while others' is thin. The muscular force with which his come is shot makes the difference in distance (if you're measuring), and some guys shoot pretty far, while with others there is no shooting going on at all.

High Tea

by Alison Tyler

4:00 p.m. Thursday. Dainty ceramic teapot nestled beneath a white crocheted warmer. Sterling silver service polished to a reflecting sheen. Antique lace tablecloth so fine it could tear if you looked at it too hard.

Last place on fucking earth you'd find my boyfriend, Charlie.

His gold-flecked eyes are wide open, and he tosses his long, glossy-black hair out of his face with an impatient shrug. "You're kidding, right?" he asks, visibly flinching when I tell him what I want.

"An array of delicacies served to us in our own suite by a private waiter well schooled in the age-old ritual of high tea," I continue, undaunted by his expression. I am repeating a passage from the slick brochure of one of San Francisco's most famous—and snobby—hotels. A passage that has turned me on indescribably.

Charlie just stares, dark brows arched incredulously. *What have I done with his girlfriend?* his expression says. *And who is this Martha Stewart–like impostor who has taken her place?*

"You won't regret it," I assure him, and he finally reads the look in my green eyes correctly, because he begrudgingly nods his okay. Promised pleasure will make people do the most unusual things.

4:15. Thursday. The tuxedoed waiter has left, and Charlie is a true believer. Fantasy feast of finger-length cucumber and cream cheese sandwiches is ignored in favor of a far more decadent fantasy. Tiny tea cakes sit iced so prettily all alone. And my man is spread out on the richly carpeted floor, tan slacks open, receiving his first time ever tea-flavored blow job.

"Oh, God, Julie. Take another sip."

The fragrant liquid fills my mouth and I hold it for a second, swishing slightly before swallowing. Then I'm back down on him, my lips hot from the Earl Grey, the welcoming sensation of a prewarmed mouth caressing his rock-hard rod. Sip, swallow, and suck. We could do this all day.

"Too good," Charlie groans and arches his slim hips, pressing forward, gaining the contact he craves. "More. Please—"

Pinkie in the air, I drink again, taking my time to savor the flavor, a combination now of the strong tea and the hot-summertime taste of my boyfriend's naked skin. I am wearing sleek white gloves and a ruffled pastel party dress in place of my standard uniform of faded Levi's, turtleneck sweater, and beat-up black leather jacket.

But my soft caramel hair has come down from its too-tight bun, and I feel that my perfectly applied lipstick has smeared. No outfit has ever excited me more.

Charlie's warm brown eyes burn me with their heat as I swallow the tea, and then he stands, strips out of his clothes, and gets ready to really play. Gripping onto my shoulders, he moves my body, so that I'm on my back and he's positioned above me, thrusting hard and slowly into my willing, waiting mouth. I look up at him, at the tribal tattoos that criss-cross his broad biceps, at the silver hoops piercing his nipples. He's comfortable cruising the steepest city hills on his Ducati. Or spread underneath his treasured old Chevy pickup with his battered toolbox nearby. He's at ease in dangerous places that would scare every upper-crust guest in this elite hotel.

And now he's turned on by teatime.

When his cock presses against the back of my throat, I reach one hand up to find his balls as he sets the rhythm of the ride. The light caress of my still-gloved fingers takes Charlie to a higher level.

"That, Julie," he whispers urgently. "Keep doing that."

My fingertips make gentle circles as my mouth sucks harder. Careful rotations of soft fabric against even softer skin. The two differing sensations make Charlie close his eyes and moan, thrusting even harder and then holding still. Sealing himself to me. I'm growing wetter beneath the silly ruffles of the dress, and I look up from my position on the floor and see pink-orange sunlight filtering through the scalloped lace edge of the tablecloth.

It's going to be a long afternoon.

Four-ish. Every Thursday. Our place.

We own our own mismatched tea service now, purchased for pennies at a second-hand store. And a small selection of teas resides in our cabinet, seemingly out of place near the bottles of exotic tequila and Johnny Walker Black Label. Charlie sets the scene himself, his large hands working to stay calm as he envisions the pleasures that await him. Delicate teacups rattle on their saucers. Petite cookies jump on the plate as he sets it onto the tray.

I put one hand on his to slow him down, and then we partake in the ritualistic and aristocratic pleasure of high tea.

3

For Him

I'm going to start this chapter, the chapter for the man who will, I hope, soon be receiving fellatio, with a broad, sweeping statement: you guys are expected to know everything. Everything, especially about sex. In our culture, men are expected to take the lead, know what to do, know how everything works, and have all the answers in bed—*not* to ask questions. Not to be filled with wonder at the mysteries of the human body and pleasure. And definitely not to explore the far reaches of your desire or push the boundaries of con- ventional male sexuality. The worst part is that there's a serious lack of ways for men to find answers, unless you know where to look. It's hard for men to even ask the questions, something that you'll eventually need to give yourself permission to do, and feel okay about. I look at how men are stereotyped, layered with expectations, and given few options, and I think that you got a raw deal. The deck is stacked against you.

Male sexuality is grossly oversimplified and stereotyped everywhere you turn. Movies, advertising, and other forms of popular culture reinforce the narrow sex box you're supposed to fit in, and most sex guides are no better. You're either one way or the other: you know all the answers and everything's okay, or you don't. You're either gay or straight, with no fuzzy lines anywhere in between. That's how we have come to see male sexuality, and if a man isn't sure about sex or wants to find out more, or maybe wants to try a sex act or idea that's outside the box, he gets labeled. The guidebooks, and practically everything else relating to men and sex, seem to be convinced that all guys want to do is "insert, thrust, repeat," and they think that to speak to men about sex they need to either use pithy, punchy sports euphemisms or employ an overly academic tone. How insulting it all is.

Sexuality is a spectrum of expression for everyone. There will always be new desires to explore and new things to investigate, try, reject, try again…

Fellatio as a sex act is deceptively simple. Just stick your dick into your partner's waiting mouth—and bam! Right? Well, not quite. There's plenty to learn about being a great receptive fellatio partner. You'll be surprised—and aroused—as you find out the many ways that you can receive pleasure through oral stimulation. So, roll up your sleeves, and dig in.

A Prelude to a Kiss

It all begins with desire. Arousal, lust, need, passion, and the specific desire to feel your partner's mouth envelop your penis and lick your testicles, scrotum, and anus. Or perhaps it's your partner's desire that's doing the talking. At some point in the erotic dance you share with your partner, you'll know that soon you will be on the receiving end of oral sex.

As they say, it takes two to tango, and you and your lover are two equal halves of the fellatio experience. When you're with a new partner experimenting with new sexual expressions (such as adding fellatio to your routine), paying attention to what's going on for both of you is crucial.

> *The first time I got head, I was utterly terrified after the first 60 seconds—not because I thought I was doing something wrong, but because it didn't feel good. I mean, it felt OK, but it wasn't the mind-blowing experience I had been led to believe it would be. As a matter of fact, I was pretty bored. I just lay there while my girlfriend went up and down methodically on my dick...and I started to lose my hard-on long before I was anywhere close to coming. I felt horrible—as if I was doing something wrong. It took me a long time to figure out that getting head is an active process— you have to stay involved with your partner, your fantasy, your erotic connection, or you just become a passive bump on a log, and that's not sexy at all.*

I'm not just talking about physical safety for you and your partner, but the emotional temperature of both participants. If you're both comfortable with fellatio, have clearly agreed to proceed, and are both fine with the sometimes fuzzy boundaries of control between giver and receiver in the fellatio exchange, then you're in great shape. But if it's your first time receiving oral sex or your partner's first time performing it, if you feel unsure or anxious about something, or if your partner is reluctant for any reason, you'll need to find out everything you can about your own physical situation, and what's going on with your partner, before you get started.

First times have that funny catch-22 of being simultaneously scary and unforgettable. With a partner who is giving fellatio for the first time, you'll want to be more supportive than you would have ever thought necessary—patience, words of encouragement, slow pacing, and the willingness to stop at any time will help ensure a first time you'll want to remember. If oral sex is something you've requested but your partner is reluctant, be aware of the pressure they may be feeling; explore their concerns in conversation, and hand them a chapter of this book to read when they need concrete answers about anything pertaining to fellatio. And understand that some people may never feel completely comfortable with fellatio, for whatever reasons, and that they will need to experience their feelings at their own pace.

> If your partner wants to perform oral sex with you, and you feel there's something bad about sex or your genitals, please tell them so they don't feel hurt by your rejection of their desires. Or if you're shy, try handing them a chapter of this book.

Perhaps you're the one stressing—about receiving oral sex. Anxiety can be no laughing matter when you're about to have a lover touch, look at, and taste your genitals. Get to the bottom of your stress by finding out what's interfering with your willingness or ability to receive pleasure. Are you unsure about the notion that your partner wants to put their face between your legs, let alone put your penis in their mouth? Take my word on it—our collective discomfort with our genitals is not limited by gender. Everyone worries about appearance, comparisons, and performance. Whether you're a newcomer or an experienced recipient of oral pleasure, you might be concerned about how you look, how you respond to the sensations, or what your partner might think about you. So get comfortable, and read on.

How Do I Look?

One absolute fact about the way men's genitals look is that every single set is different. No two penises are alike, nor do they get hard in the same way. However, the standard operating equipment is more or less the same: a penis (circumcised or not), a scrotal sack containing two testicles, and pubic hair that generally covers the mound over the pubic bone, the very base of the penis, the testicles, and the perineum (from the base of the balls to the anus). The skin on the pubic mound, the perineum, and the anus is similar in texture to the skin on the rest of the body, but usually a different shade. It deepens and changes in color as it reaches the base of the penis and the scrotum, and colors can range anywhere from light pink or peach to a tawny brown or dark chocolate. The texture is soft, and the skin is thin. If you think you may have a problem with your penis, you spot unusual bumps or lesions, there's a discharge from your urethra, you experience pain during or after sex, or your penis bends sharply upon erection, you should consult a doctor.

Penises come in a variety of shape and size combinations too vast to catalog, and there's no predicting what a soft penis will look like when erect. Long and thin, short and squat, curved up, down, left, right—it's all normal. The variations make a man average. And average size? Average depends on whose statistics you're looking at. A 1993 University of Toronto study of 63 men measured unerect penises along rulers placed at the base, and stretched them to get a range of 2 ⅜ inches to 5 ¼ inches, with 3 ¾ inches being the average. But soft

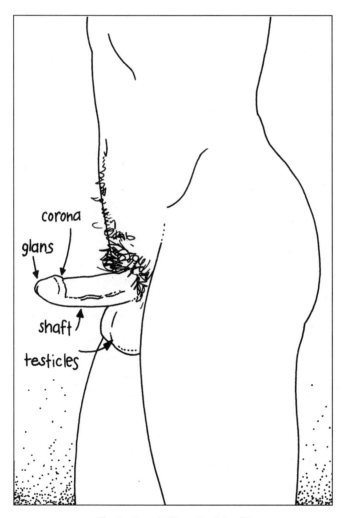

Illustration 4. How Do I Look?

means little when talking about average erect size. Almost forty years ago, Masters and Johnson found that smaller unerect penises grew more than the larger soft-ies—showing that soft penises are no barometer for size. The truth about penis size is that there's a lot of erection variation out there. But don't forget—your cock is as big as your brain, meaning that the real measure is the size of the pleasure you give (and receive).

If you want to compare how you look to men in porn movies, guys in *Playgirl,* or gay male mags, you cer-tainly can—but it won't give you an idea about what's really out there, and more important, what your part-ners are seeing. Are you worried about how you look? Do you think that your penis, testicles, anus, or pubic area are too hairy, or not enough? They don't look like the ones in porn? The cocks you see in magazines are airbrushed (often heavily) and lit, angled, covered in makeup, shaved, and positioned just *so*. In porn movies, makeup and shaving is standard, and as with the maga-zines, it's only the guys who are larger than average that make the grade. You won't see any regular penises in porn, period. And seldom any soft ones, for that matter.

The huge market for penis enlargement gadgets, injections, operations, and pills neatly serves to rein-force your insecurities and sexual shame. It's a business like any other, though it's a kissing cousin to the diet industry and the breast augmentation industry—sleazy, and offering impossibly quick fixes to get you to "fit in" to unrealistic, invented, and often impossible standards. Penis enlargement is a bad idea. Vacuum pumps work only temporarily and can cause lasting damage if used improperly; also, the erections they provide are big but soft. No pill will make your dick bigger. And remember that any surgery you have on your urogenital system will cut through nerves, fibers, and erectile tissue—things you need in order to enjoy sex. Plus, silicone implants often need to be replaced, can become infected, and look lumpy. Liposuctioned fat eventually melts back into your body. Why put yourself through any of it when you could be enjoying a blow job instead?

Do Vegetarians Taste Better?

For men who worry about odors and flavors their partners may encounter, rest assured that your genitals smell and taste exactly like you—your skin, actually. The obvious answer to any cleanliness dilemma is to shower daily, and for men who have a foreskin, to be sure to clean under the hood—any buildup will lend a funky odor. If you're wanting to impress your partner by emitting less odor, you can shower shortly before your encounter. If your partner is anxious about your flavor, showering together before fellatio can allay fears—they may even want to participate in getting you "squeaky clean" or might enjoy beginning oral sex in the tub.

If you plan to ejaculate in your partner's mouth, you might wonder if you taste okay. An obvious answer to this question is to taste it yourself first—for some, no big deal, but for others, this is something they'd rather skip. Whatever you decide, there are a few things you can do to make sure your come tastes and smells neutral. Things that can make the flavor of your semen strong or pungent are vitamins, asparagus, beets, coffee, cigarettes, and garlic. Strong substances like these can influence your ejaculate in much the same way they do your urine. To keep it smelling and tasting neutral, avoid these substances at least twenty-four hours before oral sex, and drink plenty of water. Carnivorous men tend to have stronger-tasting semen than those who stick to veg-etarian diets, though whether this is unpleasant to the person doing the tasting is debatable.

Sweetening your come is a whole different matter. Conventional wisdom on this subject (if there is such a thing) states that if you want to make your ejaculate more palatable you should drink lots of citrus, pineapple, or celery juice, and eat a lot of sweet melon. However, the jury seems to be out on the results, and it will probably be around eight hundred years before someone does a real study on the effects of cantaloupe on the taste of come.

There are a few products on the market that claim to enhance the bouquet and zest of semen, most notably Seminex and Cum-So-Sweet. Both products claim not only to make it sweeter but also to impart it with a citrus flavor that "women will love." Seminex is a powder that comes in packets; you mix it with water and drink before you go to bed for two to three days before you want to be tasty. Cum-So-Sweet is a sublin-gual tablet (it dissolves under the tongue) that both partners use just before oral sex to change the taste of whatever fluid ends up in your mouth—sadly (and mis-takenly), it's assumed by the manufacturers that pussy is also an undesirable taste and that both partners are het-erosexual. No products that make these claims have passed any sort of clinical or safety trials, so buyer beware, and read the ingredients of any product that makes these claims before you ingest it.

Erection Questions

Contrary to popular conceptions, men's erections and orgasms don't erupt like Old Faithful. Nothing in the male or female pleasure cycle is entirely predictable, and that goes for arousal, orgasm, ejaculation, the timing involved for any of it, and especially erection. Erections work on two levels simultaneously. One is the physical: touching your genitals or an erogenous zone, or having them touched, triggers a response along nerve pathways to begin the flow of blood into your penis. The other level is the path that leads directly from your brain: an image, fantasy, idea, or mental or visual stimulus triggers the same nerve response, filling your penis with blood and growing it into an erection. The stiffest cocks and the hottest sex come when both pathways are stimulated at the same time.

The perplexing thing about erections is that they sometimes like to come and go as they please. They arrive at the party uninvited or leave when everyone's having fun. During sex they'll stiffen and soften as your pleasure cycle dips and peaks along its normal course. This swelling and shrinking may not be noticeable, or it may gradually become more noticeable with age, anxiety, stress, or medication. Sometimes these issues make erections unreliable altogether.

The best course of action when you're concerned that you won't be able to achieve or sustain an erection is a piece of frustrating, though accurate, advice: relax. Stressing out about having a hard-on creates inner tension and turmoil, making it almost impossible to access the neural pathway whereby the brain engages the cock—sometimes physical stimulation can conquer the inner demons, but not always. Anxiety, anger, and guilt kill erections, period. However, if you are experiencing pain or numbing, or if you are taking medication that may effect erections or are having other health problems, talk to your doctor about what's going on. Just keep in mind that your doctor will first tell you that men with healthy erections have low-fat diets, get plenty of exercise, maintain a healthy weight, and don't smoke.

Possible Causes of Erection Difficulties

Every man is likely to have trouble achieving or maintaining an erection at some point in his life. According to the National Institutes of Health, between ten and thirty million American men have consistent trouble. Causes may include the following:

DRUGS OR MEDICATION
- Anti-anxiety meds, such as BuSpar, Valium, and Xanax
- Antidepressants, including Prozac and Zoloft
- Antifungal meds, such as Flagyl, Diflucan, and Nizoral
- High blood pressure meds, including Inderal and Lopressor
- Party drugs such as crystal meth (speed), cocaine, alcohol, ecstasy, and pot
- Drugs for substance abuse, such as Anabuse and methadone
- Ulcer meds, such as Tagamet

HEALTH CONDITIONS AND OTHER CAUSES
- Arteriosclerosis
- Diabetes
- High cholesterol/high blood pressure
- Low testosterone from age or HIV
- Neurological issues, possibly from an accident, surgery, MS, or Parkinson's disease
- Prostate problems
- Smoking
- Stress and depression

To have better, stronger, and more dependable erections, have more of them. Your penis is comprised of more than 50 percent muscle—smooth muscles, not the kind you can bulk up. In order to be healthy and function properly, this muscle tissue needs oxygen, which it gets in the form of blood that flows in when you're aroused. The best way to keep the tissue oxygenated is to include regular sexual stimulation in your daily life, such as masturbation or sex with a partner.

And while we're working on your new sexual exercise routine, don't forget to do your Kegels. Dr. Arnold Kegel was a gynecologist who taught women to strengthen their pubococcygeal (PC) muscles, initially to help with incontinence. The side effect turned out to be more (and stronger) orgasms for the women who practiced the exercises regularly. Men have the same muscles lining the pelvic floor, and when they do their Kegels, their orgasms become more powerful and last longer; some men also report a faster recovery time between erections.

To find your Kegel muscles, stop the flow of urine midstream. These are the muscles you want to flex. Do Kegels anywhere, anytime you feel comfortable. A daily routine is recommended: start by contracting the muscles for a count of three, five to ten times. Then do a series of rapid squeezes in sets of fifteen. As time goes by, you can increase your reps, and experiment with holding your contractions for longer periods of time.

Coming Too Soon

Early ejaculation is often considered the curse of young men, or men who are new to having sexual experiences. It's frustrating when it happens, even more so when you are no longer young or new to sex. In truth, it's a common thing that happens to most men, and it happens to all men at some point in their lifetime.

If you're young or new to sex, then you can rest assured that control will soon be yours with a little time and experience. If early ejaculation stems from hypersensitivity, you can use a condom or even two, and experiment with frequent masturbation to decrease your penis's sensitivity. But if you just plain keep coming before you're ready, and you've checked in with your partner and they have expressed the desire for you to last longer, you have a couple of options.

Try using the squeeze technique. This is done by placing a hand at the tip of your penis so that the thumb is on the underside, pressing on the frenulum (brush up on your anatomy in chapter 2, "The Anatomy of a Man's Pleasure"), with the fingertips placed on either side of the coronal ridge. When you feel yourself getting close to orgasm, squeeze for three or four seconds, then release. This will make your erection subside a little, and you should wait about thirty seconds before continuing with sexual stimulation. The squeeze technique can be used three or four times during your encounter, and as a delicious side effect, it will make your orgasm very powerful. Some men prefer squeezing at the base of their penis, or instead of squeezing, pulling their balls down—experiment on your own during masturbation to see what works best. Then try it with your partner; some men enjoy having their partner do the squeezing.

An alternative solution is the stop-start technique. At the same point that you would employ the squeeze technique, stop the stimulation altogether until the feeling of impending orgasm subsides. Practice this once a day, and see how long you can make the waiting period last. The more you practice, the more control you'll have over your orgasms.

> I was very close to coming, but every time I was just about to explode, she would momentarily stop her oral actions and squeeze me firmly at the base with her fingers. Over the next few minutes she performed this maneuver three more times, and I was going crazy, on the verge of coming but not. It felt sooo good.

Masturbation and Fantasy

You might have noticed that I'm enthusiastic about masturbation. Masturbation is the cornerstone of our sexuality—it's where we build our fantasies and learn how we like to be touched. Masturbation is a source of release on many levels. Unfortunately, our culture has a restrictive view of it and tends to shroud masturbation in a cloak of shame or failure—but that is changing with the times. Still, some guys might see jacking off as a negative thing: a self-defeating substitute for partnered sex, a secret shame, an admission of guilt. These ideas are damaging, and if you are coping with these feelings when you want to masturbate, consider what effect these self-deprecating thoughts may have on your emotions, and your emotional future.

It can be difficult to release guilt if your sexual fantasies are making you uncomfortable. An erotic fantasy is a thought, idea, image, or scenario that is sexually interesting to you. It doesn't have to turn you on; or it may turn you on a little, or a lot. If you think you don't fantasize, think again. Fantasies can emerge from your erotic imagination in different forms; they can be detailed or fragmented. We may see famous people that are attractive and imagine that our lives overlap. We revisit memories of times we have enjoyed, and they make us feel good in the present. Often, we envision scenarios that have never happened and some that aren't even possible. Sometimes we tell others what we have done, making a fantasy for them—or us—come true. Whatever shape your fantasies take, looking at them can open doors to understanding what arouses you and allow you to tap into new channels of erotic expression—channels that work for you.

For some people, fantasies aren't an area they care to explore. Because they come from our imagination, and therefore are connected with our subconscious, fantasies can be startling, unpredictable, and sometimes even shocking. When we become aroused it's easy to surrender ourselves to whatever movie we're running in our heads, and push it in the direction that gets us closer to orgasm—but sometimes afterward, we might realize that what got us off was beyond what we deem acceptable in our daily lives. It's easy to feel guilty after a fantasy has gone somewhere we find unpleasant or offensive. Admitting this guilt can make us feel shame about sex, our desires, or even who we are. Especially if the fantasy was powerful and included something that we would never do in real life, like degrade ourselves or betray a loved one. When fantasies move toward the arenas of everyday life (as they are bound to do), they can manifest in ways that make us uncomfortable.

Sometimes it's not the content of the fantasies that can trigger guilt, but the time and place they occur. They can happen at inconvenient times, such as at work or on the bus, placing you in a sexually charged situation in your head while the world goes on around you—this may feel inappropriate or "dirty." Or they can happen during sex with a partner; while the partner is fully present (yet unaware), you are imagining things to get yourself off from the stimulation that they provide. The illusion is created that somehow you've betrayed them. It's important to understand the role of fantasy in sex before beating yourself up about what, how, with whom, or when you fantasize.

We all know that fantasy is not reality. But when we masturbate and imagine troubling things, people, or situations, our human curiosity kicks in and we ask ourselves if these things are what we really want. For some people this is a horrifying thought. It's important to keep in mind that fantasies don't necessarily bear any relationship to reality. The realm of fantasy is the sanctuary in your mind where you are free to enjoy things that you would never do in real life. And fantasy is not only a place where we can court the forbidden but also a powerful sex toy that can be used for arousal, heightening pleasure, and achieving climax.

Think about your fantasies for a moment, whether they are vivid, vague, seemingly mundane, or a little scary. Don't try to look deeply into their meanings, just pick out their main themes. What you're doing is isolating what it is that makes them a peak erotic experience for you and mining them for their erotic potential. Keep your mind open, and reserve judgment on yourself—this isn't about "good" and "bad," it's about understanding what turns you on. Note what stands out, and the important differences between what is possible in fantasy and what is possible in reality.

Now you're getting an idea of your main fantasy components. Think about what your favorite themes are, or try on new ideas that appeal to you. Feel comfortable with tapping into what these fantasies trigger when you want to become aroused. Remember that if you fantasize about something shocking, like being forced to perform sex, it doesn't mean that you want it to happen or that you are a bad person. But by identifying it in the realm of your fantasies, you can find a safe space where imagination fuels desire. By learning how to turn yourself on with fantasy, you can do extraordinary things, such as making yourself really aroused and teaching yourself a new masturbation technique (for instance, delaying orgasm). Or you can fantasize while your partner goes down on you, and learn to orgasm with the combination of their stimulation and your fantasy. Or if you have established trust and good sexual communication with a partner, you can share your fantasies—you can even make some of them come true.

Use your fantasies freely when you masturbate, and use masturbation as a tool to learn about, explore, and enhance your own sexuality. As former U.S. Surgeon General Joycelyn Elders, M.D., said about masturbation, "It's practicing for sex." Here are some suggestions for masturbation:

- Learn your own topography. Read about your anatomy in chapter 2, "The Anatomy of a Man's Pleasure."
- Set aside some time for yourself when you have no obligations and some privacy. Treat yourself to something nice and sensual, like a relaxing shower or bath, a new lubricant, or an adult magazine or movie.
- Try masturbating in different positions. You can sit in a chair, lie on your belly or back, or visit different rooms in your house.

- Get familiar with your own touch, running your hands all over your torso, thighs, ass, and genitals. Make yourself acquainted with your cock and balls by touching them, and look at them in a mirror if you can (and if you're comfortable with this).
- Using lubricant, caress your genitals with your hands, spending time to linger in the spots that feel good. Familiarize yourself with the different skin textures and colors, and take note of your favorite spots. Circle the head with the palm of your hand, massage it making a fist, or even pinch it gently with your fingers
- Guys use vibrators, too. If you want to use a vibrator, set it on its lowest speed and run it over your thighs, on your pubic mound, and at the base of your penis. Experiment with touching your perineum, scrotum, and penis with the vibrator. Get yourself in the mood with indirect stimulation, then move the vibe where it feels best. Trust yourself.
- If you'd like to learn a different technique for masturbation or orgasm, get yourself aroused—really aroused—with your regular technique and slowly begin to introduce the new behavior. It may not catch on the first few times, but it will as you continue to incorporate it into your pleasure cycle.
- Remember to breathe! Some men tend to hold their breath as they reach orgasm, but guys who use Tantric practices say that their orgasms are more intense when they use deep breathing techniques as they masturbate. As you touch yourself, inhale deeply into your belly and imagine the breath going all the way down into your pelvis, then back out.
- Tease yourself. When something feels really good— as in, imminent-orgasm good—back off and touch

yourself somewhere else, such as your nipples. This prolongs your pleasure and can make your orgasm really intense.

• Don't be afraid to bring your techniques into your partnered encounters. It may seem a little scary at first, but most lovers will want to know what you like and will find it really exciting if you show them. Masturbating during oral sex can make for some mind-blowing encounters.

Head Etiquette

I hate it when guys are silent while I'm blowing them. I want to hear dirty talk! I don't want him to be passive.

Fellatio is really hot when both partners are actively involved. Sure, it's nice to lie back, enjoy, and relax, but there are a few things you can—and should—do to make your lover feel included and appreciated, and to help allay any fears a reluctant partner might have. Consider for a moment what your partner is encountering when they go down on you. They're going to be up close to your genitals and in a position that may feel vulnerable or even physically uncomfortable. They will be taking in a whole lot of sensory information, such as sights, sounds and—oh yes—smells, in addition to wanting to accommodate your needs, while staying comfortable in what can sometimes be cramp-inducing positions.

Before you begin, if you have the slightest inkling that you may be about to have an oral escapade, take a minute to visually inspect your genitals, and run your hands, a hairbrush, or a comb through your pubic hair to remove any strays. Taking a shower before may not be possible (unless that's part of your evening's erotic agenda), but for squeamish partners a shower or bath might be a prerequisite. If you know you really need a shower, gently let your partner know, and they'll likely be thrilled that you care about their comfort and desire enough to be aware of their experience.

Whether to spit or swallow semen is an issue that goes through the mind of everyone who goes down on a man. Some don't mind it and feel quite neutral about the topic; others enjoy the taste of a man and love to swallow. In equal measure there are people who find the concept distasteful, and for a variety of reasons: the taste, the texture, their comfort level with fellatio, their comfort with a particular person, or simply their comfort around bodily fluids in general. For some it is an act of devotion, while others don't think twice about it. It is extremely good etiquette to find out how your partner feels about you ejaculating in their mouth. If your sweetie is unsure about swallowing, let them know that you will tap their shoulder (or establish some other signal) when you are close to orgasm, so they may decide what they want to do when you ejaculate.

Fellatio as a sex act has a power dynamic implied, whether you intend it to or not. Many people see the person giving head as submissive, and the person getting head as the powerful one, the one in control. This perception comes from a number of different sources; gender stereotypes, the pure physical interpretation of the act, media portrayal of fellatio, and the fact that it is a sex act that can be forced on an unwilling partner. In established relationships (or carefully negotiated ones), there is a level of trust and communication that addresses this issue—but for a significant number of people, the power implications involved in fellatio are always present in the back of their mind. Some people feel downright uncomfortable about the surrender they feel is implicit in giving head, and they can have such powerful feelings about it that they might not want to do it at all. These feelings are especially sharp for abuse survivors.

Unless you have clearly negotiated a power-exchange dynamic, be patient and let your partner go at their own pace. Thrusting into their mouth, or grabbing their hair or the sides of their head, will freak out anyone who already feels uncomfortable about fellatio. Sometimes the feeling of being forced—even a little—can trigger strong negative emotions. You may discover that your partner enjoys this, but you must find out explicitly beforehand.

Be fully present and aware of your partner's reactions. If they gag, back off and let them take the lead. Muscle fatigue may make their tongue and mouth sore—actions of the tongue and neck require a lot of energy. It might seem frustrating to have them switch to using their hands when you are close to coming, but it's a natural part of the sex play cycle, and a momentary switch in activities or a change in position will make your orgasm all the sweeter.

Staying Safe and Getting Off

Some people think that receiving oral sex is a passive act—you just sit back and enjoy the pleasure—but it's really not. Sure, you could lie back, close your eyes, and transport yourself to a fantasy realm (nothing wrong with that), but even when you're "checked out," you still are participating as one half of a two-person sex act. It's important to keep this in mind and to have already thought about a couple of things before you engage in fellatio.

Begin by concerning yourself with safety—the safety of both yourself and your partner from sexually transmitted infections and viruses, in addition to the emotional safety of both people involved. Though in chapter 4, "Know the Hard Facts: Health Considerations," I go into detail about safer sex during fellatio, you should know that fellatio, when performed to ejaculation, is considered an activity that puts both parties at moderate risk. Fellatio without ejaculation is in the low-risk category, though it's possible that you could pick up a virus if your partner has cuts or sores in their mouth.

One way to approach safer sex is to think about it as a process of trying your best to make informed choices about sex. Just as with any potentially risky act—a risky move on the freeway, giving your phone number to someone you just met—making an informed decision about sex acts requires that we know the risks we are taking when we choose to do these things.

The fact of the matter is that if you are unprotected, you are at risk for sexually transmitted diseases. If your partner has mouth sores or tiny cuts from having recently brushed or flossed their teeth, then the risk is increased—for both of you. If your partner has a viral STD such as herpes, or HPV, you can be infected by receiving a blow job without a condom. (There is a small chance you could be infected with hepatitis C this way, too.) And if you have an STD, such as HPV, hepatitis C, or HIV, you can infect your partner through unprotected fellatio. It is essential to use protection—latex or nonlatex condoms—if either of you has a viral STD. But be sure that you don't use animal-skin condoms, such as lambskin, for safer-sex protection of any kind; they won't keep you safe.

Similarly, bacterial STDs, such as chlamydia and syphilis, can be transmitted through unprotected fellatio. Both the person giving fellatio and the person receiving are at risk, though the risk level is very low. If one of you has a bacterial infection, such as chlamydia, it's a good idea to use barriers until you've completed treatment.

Some STDs can remain dormant for as long as a few years, so it's possible to give someone something you didn't even know you had. Add to all this the fact that conventional medical wisdom on safer sex and transmission of viruses and bacteria is subject to change, and can change often. Whenever in doubt, check with your doctor and keep abreast of new information by keeping up with the Centers for Disease Control, who conveniently have an STD section on their Web site, updated whenever there is new information (see chapter 13, "Resources," for contact information).

Know the Hard Facts: Health Considerations

The human body is a complex container for water, salt, sinews, bones, brains, feelings, dreams. The many things we can do with it are astounding: making buildings, babies, ideas, orgasms. The body itself is a fortress against intruders; white blood cells, helpful bacteria, and acids—nature's polymorphous armies—can combat the common cold, keeping our delicate system in balance. And yet, when compromised, our own helpful tools can be turned against us and we suddenly become the perfect host to bugs, germs, diseases, and infections. In the realm of sex, becoming a good host means anything from engaging in unprotected sex to weakening yourself with illness and uninformed lube and toy practices, all the way to being a careless (or unknowing) carrier of unfriendly bugs.

Is Fellatio Risky?

When it comes to unprotected fellatio, everyone involved is taking a risk of some kind. Unprotected fellatio carries a lower risk for the transmission of sexually transmitted diseases (STDs) than unprotected vaginal and anal intercourse (with a penis or a just-shared, unprotected sex toy), or unprotected cunnilingus (unless she ejaculates in your mouth), but there is risk involved—for both the giving and the receiving partner. When a guy gets a blow job without a condom from a stranger, he's in the low-risk category for HIV and hepatitis B and C; but he's at high risk for herpes, syphilis, gonorrhea, and HPV (human papillomavirus, or genital warts). If you go down on a man and you don't know whether he is infected, you put yourself at risk for hepatitis B, herpes, syphilis, gonorrhea, and HPV—and if you have a cut, bite, sore, or abrasion in your mouth, you are also at risk for HIV and hepatitis C. Unprotected rimming (oral-anal sex) puts you at risk for all of the above, along with hepatitis A. Brushing or flossing your teeth or going to the dentist before a round of oral sex will put you at significant risk; these activities produce tiny cuts on the gums.

Risk Awareness

Please note that the best way to avoid transmission of most viruses and STDs is to use a latex or nonlatex (but non-animal-skin) barrier for all activities involving fluid transmission.

The following tables show at a glance the risks that accompany fellatio and other sexual activities; for more details on the risks for specific STDs, see the section that follows.

Is Rimming Risky?

Rimming, or *analingus,* refers to caressing or penetrating your lover's anal opening with your tongue. Because the delicate pucker of the anus is rife with sensitive nerve endings, rimming feels incredibly pleasurable to many people, and just as many people enjoy giving it as getting it. For both givers and receivers, rimming sets the night on fire.

Though rimming is certainly enjoyable, it isn't a very safe activity. Unprotected rimming can transmit hepatitis A, anal herpes, anal warts, and possibly viruses such as HIV. Always use a barrier for rimming—but if you insist on barrier-free rimming, get a hepatitis A shot. Read about erotic rimming techniques in chapter 10, "More Techniques."

STDs and Fellatio

Some STDs are easier to transmit than others. Let's look at the most common STDs and their relative risks for transmission during fellatio.

HIV

HIV is transmitted when the blood of an infected person enters another person's bloodstream via an open cut, sore, or blood vessel. According to the Centers for Disease Control, HIV has also been found in varying amounts in semen, vaginal fluid, breast milk, and precome. The CDC cautions against allowing the blood of an infected person to make contact with mucous membranes. If you perform unprotected fellatio, you may be at risk, especially if you have a cut or sore on your lips or in your mouth (perhaps from recently brushing or flossing your teeth). While great strides have been made

Fellatio (Giving)

HIGH RISK	MODERATE RISK	NO RISK	N/A
Gonorrhea	Chlamydia	Hepatitis A	Bacterial vaginosis
Hepatitis B	Hepatitis C		Vaginitis
Herpes	HIV		
HPV	Lice/scabies		
Syphilis			

Fellatio (Getting)

HIGH RISK	MODERATE RISK	NO RISK	N/A
Gonorrhea	Chlamydia	Hepatitis A	Bacterial vaginosis
Hepatitis B	Hepatitis C		Vaginitis
Herpes	HPV		
Syphilis	HIV		
	Lice/scabies		

Rimming (Getting)

HIGH RISK	MODERATE RISK	NO RISK	N/A
Gonorrhea	Chlamydia	Hepatitis A	Bacterial vaginosis
Hepatitis B	Hepatitis C		Vaginitis
Herpes	HPV		
Syphilis	HIV		
	Lice/scabies		

Rimming (Giving)

HIGH RISK	MODERATE RISK	NO RISK	N/A
Gonorrhea	Chlamydia	None	Bacterial vaginosis
Hepatitis A	Hepatitis C		Vaginitis
Hepatitis B	HIV		
Herpes	Lice/scabies		
HPV			
Syphilis			

Sharing Sex Toys

HIGH RISK	MODERATE RISK	NO RISK	N/A
Chlamydia	Bacterial vaginosis	None	None
Gonorrhea	Hepatitis A		
Hepatitis B	Hepatitis C		
HIV	Herpes		
Syphilis	HPV		
	Lice/scabies		
	Vaginitis		

Deep Kissing

HIGH RISK	MODERATE RISK	NO RISK	N/A
None	Gonorrhea	Chlamydia	Bacterial vaginosis
	Hepatitis B	Hepatitis A	Vaginitis
	Herpes	Hepatitis C	
	HPV	HIV	
	Syphilis	Lice/scabies	

Dry Kissing

HIGH RISK	MODERATE RISK	NO RISK	N/A
None	None	Bacterial vaginosis	None
		Chlamydia	
		Gonorrhea	
		Hepatitis A	
		Hepatitis B	
		Hepatitis C	
		Herpes	
		HIV	
		HPV	
		Lice/scabies	
		Syphilis	

in managing HIV infection, there is no cure for HIV. The virus can lie dormant in the body for a very long time and can be transmitted even when there are no symptoms present. The person infected with HIV may not even know they have it.

Hepatitis

Hepatitis A, B, and C infect millions of people worldwide and can be asymptomatic for years before liver disease is evident. Hepatitis A is transmitted through oral-fecal contact and can be contracted when rimming an unprotected partner (for more on rimming, see the section above). Hepatitis B is very similar in transmission to HIV: it is found in blood and other body fluids, such as semen, vaginal secretions, breast milk, and tears. You contract hepatitis B when fluids from a carrier, such as pre-come or ejaculatory fluid, enter your body via an opening such as a cut or sore in your mouth. Hepatitis C is found only in the blood of an infected partner. That doesn't mean, however, that you shouldn't treat it like any other serious virus, and if you think your partner might be infected you should follow safer-sex guidelines at all times when performing fellatio. Hepatitis A has no chronic or long-term infection; there is a vaccine to prevent both hepatitis A and B, and they can be can be treated in some cases; there is no cure or vaccine for hepatitis C.

Herpes

Herpes is an extremely contagious STD. There are basically two types of herpes—oral and genital—and what lives in the mouth can easily take up residence in the genitals. Herpes is spread when sores or shedding skin from an infected partner make contact with mucous membranes—penis to mouth and mouth to penis—as well as through skin-to-skin contact, such as hand-to-penis or hand-to-anus contact. That's why you should use gloves with your condoms—fellatio is almost always a hands-on activity, and you'll definitely want to touch your partner's penis, balls, and/or anus while going down on him. While it's true that the herpes virus is benign when not active, the CDC states that it's possible to contract herpes between eruptions, when the skin is shedding (before an outbreak). An outbreak can range from a collection of blistering, painful sores to one small sore that can be unknowingly tucked in a fold of skin. There is no cure for herpes.

HPV

Human papillomavirus (HPV) is the virus associated with genital warts. However, you can have HPV and never have a genital wart; in fact, most people who have HPV do not know they have it, because it usually causes no symptoms. Approximately ten of the thirty identified strains of HPV can lead to the development of cervical cancer in women. HPV is spread much like herpes, through skin-to-skin and mucous membrane contact when the virus is apparent or simply shedding. It should be considered highly contagious, and you are at much higher risk for contracting HPV through fellatio than you are for contracting HIV or hepatitis. The symptoms of HPV can take several weeks or even months to appear, if they appear at all. They can be small, painless bumps or look like a collection of cauliflower-like constellations, appearing on the penis, scrotum, thighs, mouth, anus, or vagina. Again, gloves and condoms are advised, but if you see symptoms you'll want to avoid sexual contact until the outbreak has cleared up, since HPV is spread by touch and can appear in areas condoms don't cover. There is no cure for HPV.

Bacterial STDs

Gonorrhea, chlamydia, and syphilis are bacterial STDs that are spread through unprotected sexual contact. You are at much more at risk of contracting gonorrhea or syphilis through fellatio than you are of contracting HIV or hepatitis. Though transmission of chlamydia through fellatio is unlikely, it has been shown to appear in the throat. Unless you and your partner have been tested for chlamydia (which usually has no symptoms or looks like mild gonorrhea or a yeast infection), it's safest to use condoms. Gonorrhea can be spread via unprotected oral contact, as can syphilis if there is a sore (chancre) present on your mouth or his penis. These STDs can be treated with antibiotics, but if left undetected they can become serious.

Safer Sex

Sexually transmitted diseases can remain dormant for months or even years after exposure, so it's possible to pass on something you didn't even know you had. This is why it's essential to use barriers—latex or non-latex—when coming in contact with a partner's sexual fluids.

If either you or your partner has an STD, safer-sex practices are *required* to prevent transmission. If one of you has a viral STD, such as hepatitis C, HIV, HPV, or herpes, use latex (or non-latex, such as nitrile or polyurethane, but not animal skin, such as lambskin condoms—see "Condoms" below for more information) barriers during fellatio. It may also be helpful to talk to your physician or an STD prevention specialist (see chapter 13, "Resources," for hotlines and organizations) about the risks for transmission in your particular case.

If one of you has a bacterial infection such as chlamydia, you *must* use barriers until you've completed treatment. If you have a cut or bite in your mouth, the risk to both partners is greatly increased. Keep this in mind if you've recently brushed or flossed your teeth, both of which can cause tiny cuts and bleeding in your mouth. Don't despair—there are many options out there for the orally inclined apprentice who wants to stay safe.

However, not everyone who comes to the fellatio table needs to use a barrier. Once you and your partner have been tested for all STDs and are sure you are free from infection, you may decide to have sex only with each other. Or you may choose to become *fluid bonded,* a term that means the parties involved have had updated tests for STDs and infections and have explicitly agreed to have unprotected sex only with each other and use barriers with all other partners.

We all make our own choices about everyday risks, and most of them are informed—we know the risks involved in smoking, walking down a dark street at night alone, or having a one-night stand with a stranger. Life is full of these decisions. With sex, the important thing is to understand that safer sex involves a spectrum of choices and is not an either/or issue. We determine what safer-sex practices we are comfortable with and what our acceptable levels of risk are, and we each make our own set of safer-sex "rules." For instance, some possible rules are "no fellatio from strangers without a condom" or "unprotected oral sex only with my partner." This way, we choose the risks we take. And since we're human and love to make rules and then break them, we can also examine what might cause us to break those rules; perhaps alcohol, drugs, trust issues, love—or fear of judgment.

Risk assessment is the process of honestly assessing your own risky sexual behaviors, such as preferring unprotected fellatio or engaging in unprotected intercourse, and determining how risky they are. It's also assessing the risk level of your potential partners. For instance, if a partner has been recently tested (and they are free from STDs), they can be considered a low-risk partner for unprotected sex, but if you enjoy unprotected oral sex on the first date, then your partners may be high-risk. And having this type of sex with them puts you in the high-risk category, too.

Safer Sex Made Easy: Gear

Safer sex is a term usually associated with using condoms for intercourse or fellatio with a new partner to prevent transmission of STDs or pregnancy. But the applications for the many types of safer-sex gear currently available go much further than making certain types of sex safer. Even if you're in a long-term, monogamous relationship, you'll be surprised at just how useful safer-sex gear is for adding pleasure and spontaneity (yes, spontaneity!) to your oral adventures. Plus, there are some safer-sex items that you will always want to have handy: gloves serve a dual purpose of preventing the spread of certain bacteria and facilitating cleanup in a snap, while a selection of unlubricated condoms can make your insertable sex toys ready to use without a trip to the sink to clean them.

For fellatio or rimming, you can choose among different types of protection to suit your individual style and preferences, or you can tailor them to make a specific encounter sizzle. The thought of a mouthful of latex may seem unappealing to you, or not as intimate as you like, but I encourage you to consider the risks and make an informed decision. When you decide which methods you want to use, set aside some time alone to taste, smell, examine, and handle the items before you put them to use.

Condoms

> I've only gone down on five guys, but I have to admit that I never thought once about using a condom.

> I love sucking guys off when they have condoms on: I don't have to worry about what to do when they come.

Before you put anything in your mouth, you really should know where it's been first. But when knowing is just not possible, and that thing you want in your mouth is a penis or strap-on, then what you need is a condom.

Condoms prevent many STDs from making you their next home; when used properly, they've been shown to prevent transmission of most viruses and infections. You don't want a hot round of fellatio to become a bittersweet memory of the times before you caught X, Y, or Z—so find some latex or nonlatex condoms that you don't mind tasting while wrapping your lips around your favorite lollipop.

Unlubricated condoms are the best to have around for giving head, mainly because they're not coated with that vile-tasting lube that lubricated condoms are marinated in. Additionally, that prepackaged lube almost always has silicone in it, which not only tastes disgusting but is also hard to get out of your mouth and can ruin some silicone dildos. Skip the lubed brands if you can, and head for the plain. Never use oil-based lubricants, massage oils, Vaseline, or anything that contains oil in conjunction with a condom. When oil touches latex, it breaks the latex down in seconds, destroying your condom, glove, dam or finger cot. Most unlubricated condoms are manufactured for oral sex, and some lubricated ones come in a plethora of fruity flavors, but you can find them unflavored: straight, no chaser. It's also important to note that animal-skin condoms (lambskin) do not prevent the transmission of viruses. Avoid them.

RECOMMENDED CONDOMS FOR FELLATIO, UNLUBRICATED

- Durex Clear Unlubricated are as straightforward as it gets. Cream-colored, reservoir tip, average length (7.5 inches), width (2.5 inches), and thickness.
- Ria colored condoms are your basic unlubricated condoms, but they come in pretty colors to make your party more festive. Reservoir tip, average length, width, thickness.
- Trojan Enz unlubricated are another stalwart friend: simple yet eloquent in cream-colored, reservoir tip, and average everything.
- Trojan Non Lube are a special breed, and a favorite for fellatio aficionados. The last of their kind, they have a plain rounded end instead of a reservoir tip that makes transmitting subtle sensations to the head of his penis effortless. Cream-colored; longer than average.

CONDOMS, FLAVORED

- Durex Flavored are a jaunty European import and were the first condom to have flavored lubricant FDA approved. Bright colors signal Carmen Miranda's favorite flavors: banana, orange, and strawberry.
- Kiss of Mint (Lifestyles) are the most popular condoms for oral sex. Thinner than most condoms, they have an extremely flared shape that makes them wider at the tip—something men really like, because it gives them more sensation. Slightly shorter than most, cream-colored, flavored with a minty powder (unlubricated), reservoir tip.
- Trustex Flavored are also FDA approved, and they turn heads by being a bit longer, wider across, and made with thinner latex than average condoms. Colorful and flavorful in strawberry, vanilla, chocolate, grape, banana, and cola. Now, if they could just add bubble gum, in pink…

CONDOMS, NONLATEX

- Avanti Polyurethane beat the pants off latex by being twice as thin and strong as a latex condom. Many people without latex sensitivities prefer Avantis for oral sex because they have no taste. Hypoallergenic and available in Super Thin, this is the widest condom available and one of the shortest (flared at the end; snugger at the base). Lubricated, and because it's not latex you don't have to worry about contact with oils.
- Trojan Supra are the second polyurethane condom to hit the market. Made of Trojan's Microsheer, they're ultra-thin, really soft in texture, and hypoallergenic, and they have no taste or smell. Like

any other superhero, they're also truly invisible. Quite wide and long, but they have a band at the base to make them stay put. The catch? Currently only available lubricated with the skin-irritating (and mouth-numbing) spermicide nonoxynol-9. Bad Trojan!

When using a condom for oral sex, you can apply it to your lover either manually (very sexy) or orally (even sexier). For the hands-on approach, first open and unroll the condom a tiny bit so you can see which way it's unrolling. Take a moment to drip a drop of lube into the very tip of the condom. The slippery surface will transmit more sensation to the head of his cock, helping him to feel every little lick. Pinch the tip, to keep the air out as you place the condom on the tip of his penis. This will make room in the condom for semen when he comes. Firmly wrap your thumb and forefinger around the base of the condom while holding the condom's tip, and unroll. It will take a few strokes to roll it down to the base, but he probably won't mind.

I'll never forget the first time I put a condom on him with my mouth! He thought it was the sexiest thing he'd ever seen, and the blow job was his favorite.

Oral application takes a little practice, but it's worth it. Place a little lube on your lips (or lick them), and suck the reservoir tip into the opening of your mouth, so the roll of the condom makes a ring around the outside of your lips. Make sure you have the inside of the condom facing out, so it will roll down over the penis. With your lips slightly parted, suck the tip of the condom in slightly and give the tip of his cock a nuzzling kiss with your lips, letting them glide down over the head. Hold the shaft with one hand, keep suction on the condom, and wrap your lips firmly over your teeth, squeezing the condom between your mouth and his penis. Push with your mouth in one smooth motion down the shaft, letting your lips unroll the condom as he goes into your mouth. It may take a few rolls. Don't worry if you can't go all the way, because your hand is there to help you finish if you need it. Because the first few tries may be awkward, it's highly recommended that you practice your technique on a dildo. Unless, of course, you have a willing partner for some potentially humorous—but very hot—erotic experiments.

Gloves

Latex and nonlatex gloves are your best friends when you want to incorporate your hands into oral sex. The feel of smooth, slippery latex fingers caressing a penis or penetrating an anus is a sensation some men go crazy for. Plus, gloves instantly solve the problem of rough hands, jagged fingernails, or hangnails. Using a glove is a good safer-sex practice, as you may have tiny cuts on your fingers you may not be aware of, and some viral STDs, such as herpes, can be transmitted by skin-to-skin contact.

Even if you are fluid bonded, you may still want to use gloves to touch his penis or for penetration. They facilitate easy cleanup: you have a messy lube-covered glove and you want to switch activities or cuddle—ta-da! You remove the glove. Without the glove, you would be washing up in the bathroom. Gloves are essential for preventing the spread of germs from your unwashed hands to his genitals, and vice-versa.

Finger Cots

You can find singular little finger condoms called finger cots at your local pharmacy (made to protect fingers with cuts, these are used a lot in restaurants). Finger cots are great for fingers that may enjoy traveling southward during a blow job (for a little penetration), and they're very discreet. They're inexpensive, indispensable, and fit easily in pockets or purses.

Dental Dams

If neither of you have latex sensitivities, you can use dental dams, or lollyes, for rimming. Dental dams are small squares of latex that are used in dentistry to isolate a tooth. They can transmit the sensations of rimming well when both sides are lubricated. Dental dams are on the thick side—thicker than a condom—so the sex industry has answered back with thinner, larger squares of latex. Glyde Lollyes are thin 10-by-6-inch sheets that come in both flavored and unflavored versions. Lixx are even thinner, but smaller (5-by-5-inch) and also come in flavored or plain versions. If you can't find dams, you can cut open a latex or nonlatex condom or glove.

The best way to use dental dams and other, smaller barriers is to first mark the "mouth" side of your barrier with a pen (one side for your mouth, the other for the anus, in case it slips or slides), then apply a drop or two of water-based lube to the recipient's anus. Press the barrier in place, and you're all set. That little dental dam can be slippery when wet, so be sure to hold it in place with your hands. Remember to switch dams when switching activities or partners.

Plastic Wrap

Latex allergies are no fun, and they can rear their ugly heads as rashes, chronic infections, or severe allergic reactions leading to anaphylactic shock. When in doubt, use plastic wrap (a.k.a. Saran Wrap) for rimming; it does the trick nicely and has playful advantages. It can be even better than those slippery little dental dam squares, because you can use long sheets of it, see through it, and even make a stay-put lickable barrier out of it! For a long time, safer-sex literature insisted on nonmicrowaveable plastic wrap, because the microwaveable variety has microscopic holes to keep your soup from exploding in the microwave. But recent research has shown that those holes don't really open up until the temperature reaches microwave oven levels—that is to say, much hotter than you're both likely to get. Still, it never hurts to be extra safe, so if you're shopping for plastic wrap for safer-sex purposes, do choose the nonmicrowaveable kind.

The Eroticism of Safer Sex

For some of us, the snap of the glove, the unfurling of a dental dam, or the tearing open of the condom package means one delicious thing: we are about to have sex. While others hem and haw about the extra steps required by safer-sex gear, or the hassle, or the lessening of sensation, we smell the latex and know we are about to "get done"—and get done *right*. It means not only that our partner is considerate and cares enough about our health to take the lead but also that we can relax and anticipate good sex, because we know we are in the hands of someone who knows a thing or two about sex. I don't know about you, but when the gloves go on

I think of a smooth and slippery hand, and I purr. Especially if they're put on with a wicked smile. And when a dam is dangled knowingly before my eyes, or a condom pack seductively slipped to me when I'm slipping lower and lower… my sexy partner is telling me there is no escape from pleasure now—and I melt.

Introducing safer-sex gear into your erotic repertoire may seem awkward or even embarrassing at first, but you'll quickly overcome these feelings by spending a little time experimenting with the new accessories. Buy some condoms, dental dams, gloves, and finger cots, and examine them when you get home. Open the packages—touch the items, feel the surface texture, pull and tug on them. Bring the items to your face and lips: become familiar with them by smelling and tasting them. Try on a glove, a finger cot. Taste a condom. Try it out with a dildo (or cucumber). Lubricate one side of a dental dam, place the lubed side on the palm of your hand, and give it a few test licks, varying the sensation to get an idea of what's in store for your lover. Most of all, begin to put your safer-sex gear in the same mental category as your sex toys—because that's what they are.

Allow latex barriers into your erotic fantasies. Incorporate them into your masturbation sessions. Imagine the naughty but sweet ways you can add them to your encounters, such as having a folded condom tucked in your garter belt or the top of your boot, or gloves conveniently placed in the pocket of your jeans.

Hair and Hygiene

Encountering our lovers, for the first time or the hundredth, means encountering them fully; taste, smell, appearance, skinny legs and all. When you go down on a guy, you're up close and personal with all these things. His pubic hair and how he wears it, how he smells and tastes are variables that depend on biology or mood. If it's your first time going down, you may be wondering just what to expect, both visually and orally. Shaved, furry, musky, or squeaky clean, men are delightful and delicious in all their permutations, and the permutations can be many.

His Pubic Hair

My ex-girlfriend and I decided to completely shave our privates. Talk about arousing experiences...

After I shaved completely (including the twins, basically everything down there), she proceeded to give me what I would consider the best blow job I've ever received. She totally loved having no hair to bother her, so she went at me with every-thing, licking up and down my shaft, licking my balls, taking me in as deep as she could...

Pubic hair is something that simply can't be avoided, no matter how polite the company or skilled the waxer. Adult men have hair that covers their pubic bone, sur-rounds the base of their penis, and continues over their testicles and scrotum—for starters. Some men are very furry and thickly carpeted; others may have a light coat-ing. It's not uncommon for guys to have a "treasure trail" of hair from their navel to the thicker patch at the pubic bone, to have hair on the base of their penis, and to have pubic hair overflowing onto their thighs. And everyone has hair in the crack of their ass—it's time we all faced this fact. Don't go by what you have seen in porn; porn stars and men in erotic magazines routinely trim and shave their pubic hair, just as the women do.

How guys wear their pubic hair is a matter of indi-vidual preference—a combination of what they want to show their lovers, what their partners prefer, and what feels most comfortable. Some guys might want to shave or trim their pubic hair to foster a neat appearance, some might like the feel of less hair, and others may do it for more sensual purposes, such as increasing skin-to-skin contact during sex.

Shaving may seem like a daunting or even scary proposition for men who have never tried it, but many men who shave love the sensitivity it affords, and the way their bare skin can feel every little touch and kiss. Men new to shaving will want to read about it before they try it. Keep in mind that a newly shaved area itches when the hair grows back in. This can be irritating, in that the itching will sometimes happen when you really can't scratch, but if you continue to shave, you will itch less as time goes by. Another thing to consider is that a

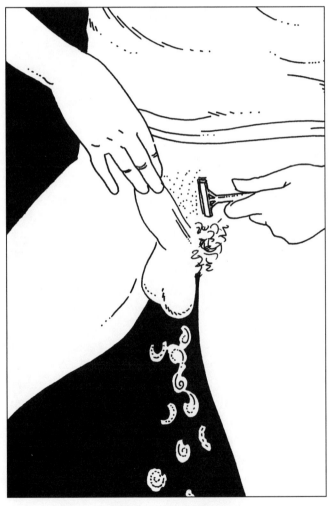

Illustration 5. Shaving

shaved area will soon become an area with stubble. The best recourse for avoiding beard burn from your pubic region on a lover's face is to either cover the stubble with a small towel or cover your pubic bone with your hand when your partner goes down on you—or shave again!

How to Shave or Trim

If you'd like to shave, follow these suggestions:
- Before starting, trim the hair down with a pair of small scissors, such as mustache trimmers, a pair of shears, or clippers.
- Take a shower or a warm bath to soften the hair.
- To decrease irritation, you might want to rub a bit of oil into the skin under the hair before shaving; try almond or olive.
- Put hair conditioner in your pubic hair even before applying the shaving cream. Hair conditioner is what's in those creams sold in adult bookstores specifically for pubic hair shaving, so you can avoid spending the extra money by getting a regular conditioner at the drugstore. Buyer beware—just use conditioner.
- Lather up well with a shaving cream or gel—a thick gel is recommended.
- Use disposable razors; you might even use two or three in a session.
- Start shaving in the same direction as the hair grows, if you can tell. The idea is to shave with as few strokes as possible. Rinse the razor in warm water after each pass; never dry shave.
- Use a mirror and sit on a towel (if you're by yourself). A chair and a full-length mirror are ideal.
- To shave the testicles and scrotum safely, stretch the skin out flat with your hand.

- When finished, rinse off using a gentle soap, pat dry, and apply a scent-fee, hypoallergenic lotion.
- Never powder! It dries out your tender, newly shaved skin. If you must dust afterward to feel dry, use only cornstarch. Of particular interest to men with female lovers, many body powders contain talc, which has been linked to cervical cancer in women.
- Yes, it can itch like crazy when it grows back in. To avoid embarrassing moments in the elevator, apply more of the hypoallergenic lotion. It won't make the itching stop forever, but it helps.

Razor Burn

Nothing's worse than making yourself lovely with a clean shave, and then having it ruined by razor burn. That uncomfortable, ugly red rash of bumps is troublesome, but it can be avoided to some extent by following the shaving suggestions presented above. If you seek further help, beware of over-the-counter and prescription creams, because they contain cortisone. Cortisone will get rid of your razor burn, but using it more than twice a week causes thinning of the skin. Try these suggestions instead:

- Splash with cool water after shaving to close your pores.
- Wash shaved areas with goat milk soap, which restores the skin's natural mantle and pH.
- Use calendula creams or ointments after shaving. Calendula works wonders on irritated skin.
- Use a natural aftershave from a health food store.
- You can find products that work well for razor bumps at drugstores (such as Tend Skin), but they usually contain harsh chemicals. Use these sparingly.

Waxing—For Men?

Yes, Virginia, men *do* get waxed. Salons that wax tend to have a client base that is both male and female, and if you think the men are only there to have their backs or chests depilated, think again. Some men do it for their partners, or for modeling or appearance concerns, and some do it for sports such as swimming or bodybuilding—so they say. Guys can and do have their bikini area waxed, and some go for the gold and get their entire genital area waxed. If you tend to get ingrown hairs, it's best to stay away from waxing, which makes hairs split and loop around under the skin's surface.

Waxing is the procedure in which a warm wax specifically formulated for hair removal is applied to the area of unwanted hair, then gauze is pressed onto it while it's still warm. When it's set, it's ripped away from the skin, taking the offending hair with it. It hurts when it's ripped away, and leaves you red and swollen for a day or two afterward. But when you consider that you're left hairless for upward of six weeks, skipping a day or two of bicycle riding isn't such a bad trade-off. Waxing can be done at home, but for delicate genital areas, you're better off putting your gonads in the hands of trained professionals.

The type of wax treatment that removes all hair in the pubic region (mound, penis, testicles, perineum, and anus) is called a "Brazilian wax." The popularity of this procedure has made it readily available in many salons, but you'll want to call around and ask a few questions before you make an appointment. Look for higher-end salons; though they cost more, it's worth it to know you're in expert hands. Find out if they wax men, because some salons cater to women only or give

Brazilians only to women. Next, find out how long their staff has been giving Brazilian waxes, specifically the staff member they will book your appointment with. Don't settle for someone who has done Brazilians for less than a year or has little experience waxing men.

When you go in to get a Brazilian, check your shyness at the door with your coat and hat. Prepare yourself to strip down in front of the cosmetologist and spread your legs into a wide, Yoga-like position. You may wind up holding your legs over your head. Be sure to go in with enough hair to wax off; if you've shaved recently, the cosmetologist might tell you to come back when your hair has grown in more. The waxing begins with a dusting of baby powder and continues with a quick slathering of wax. Even more quickly, the wax comes off, and the sensation may make you see stars. Then, a once-over with tweezers, and, well, let's hope the endorphins have kicked in, because you'll be red, swollen, and quite sore. Be prepared for the possibility of getting an unintentional erection during the process, and consider that you might have a similar arousal reaction afterward, as the pain may stimulate your blood flow and nerve endings. Any waxer who has waxed a man has seen it all before, so if you feel ashamed or embarrassed, don't sweat it—if you don't, they won't. If your doctor says it's okay with for you to take Ibuprofen, a few tablets half an hour before your wax will help minimize swelling. But the whole procedure is over in about fifteen minutes and leaves you sporting a silky-smooth cock, balls, and butt.

Aromas and Flavors

Sight, sound, touch, smell, and taste are the sensual tools with which we fully meet our world, including our lovers.

A nuzzle, an intake of breath, a caress with your lips, or the taste of a kiss all combine to filter your lover through your senses into a delicious sensory cocktail—ideally, one that is an aphrodisiac. Kisses, anywhere they land, draw your senses into erotic focus and make the pursuit of your lover's essence into passion, desire, and need. The smell, taste, and feel of a first kiss can be unforgettable.

If a kiss can be a long drink of water for our senses, then performing oral sex is like swimming in your partner's taste and scent. Erotic writings contain countless allegories that commemorate, or denigrate, the unique smells and tastes found in breeches and under skirts— yet when you're wondering just what you'll encounter when you go down on a guy, this is no help. People who love to give head will go on about how great guys taste and how much it turns them on, while others new to the game may be scared senseless about how things might taste or smell. A man's scent and taste can vary depending on any number of factors, from whether he's showered lately to whether he smokes.

But the reality is that he's going to taste and smell like whatever he tastes and smells like all over—just a little more musky. His cock may taste lightly salty or even a bit tangy, and some men exude a very faint odor of come. The taste of pre-come, the slippery substance that some men ooze from their urethral opening, can range from no flavor at all to a slight sharpness or saltiness, or it can taste like a mild version of his ejaculate. Strong foods such as asparagus or garlic can influence the urethral environment, and so can vitamins. Even if they seem undetectable, the flavors and smells from a man's genitals are packed with chemicals and pheromones that make a powerful biochemical aphrodisiac. However, this doesn't mean that his chemistry will "click" with yours, or that your lover will have the same sweet taste every time. Should you notice a marked change in his aroma or flavor, and you have both established trust in the area of oral sex, you might gently bring it to his attention, as it may warrant a health check.

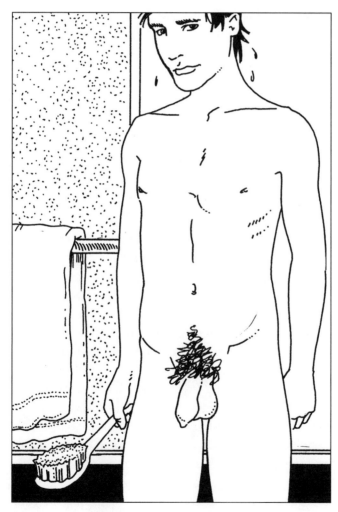

Illustration 6. Soap Him Up

If you are concerned about cleanliness, or about your own reactions to tasting or smelling him for the first time, try showering together beforehand or taking a sensual bath. This way, you can seductively soap him up, getting him thoroughly clean (and thoroughly aroused). In the bath or shower, testing out the way he feels on your lips and tongue might be easier, because you have control over both the environment and the cleanliness issue. Plus, tenderly washing and kissing him is incredibly intimate, and just plain sexy.

A Taste of Honey

> I've always been the type of girl to never swallow it. But I do with my new lover. I don't know what's different, maybe because I'm with someone I'm so crazy about that I want all of him!

If you put a man's penis in your mouth with the intention of giving him pleasure, chances are good that he's going to have an orgasm—in, or near, your mouth. How you feel about this depends on many factors; whether you enjoy the idea, the time and place of the blow job, how much you like him, or even how your relationship is going. If you don't know him, or his sexual history, then spitting or swallowing is also a question of assessing risk: semen has been shown to contain HIV, which can be dangerous if you have any tiny cuts, sores, or bites in your mouth. Somewhere between thinking you might want to go down on him and his orgasm, you're going to need to decide exactly what you're comfortable with in terms of his ejaculation. Are you okay with him coming in your mouth, or not?

The consistency and amount of come expelled upon orgasm varies from man to man. While the average amount is between one and two teaspoonfuls, some men may have close to the two teaspoons or more, while others have very little at all. The amount, texture, or flavor of a man's come has absolutely nothing to do with how powerful or pleasurable his orgasm is. One guy may have thin, watery come, while another's is thick like egg whites, or it can be anywhere in between.

Taste is another variable, and besides any dietary influences, each man is different; you may find you enjoy the flavor of one lover's come and not another's. Male ejaculate measures in at an alkaline pH of 8 (more alkaline than spit, tears, or sweat), approximately the same pH of an egg white. It can taste neutral, slightly salty, bitter, a little sweet, similar to an oyster, like a delicate Brie cheese, or even slightly tart. Many people also report very slight (though sometimes strong) odors of bleach or mushrooms. Of course, his ejaculate is going to taste and smell just like his very own brand of ejaculate, and there's only one way to find out if it's to your liking.

The taste of a man being subject to the individual's erotic palate, many fellatio fans enjoy the taste of come and like its distinctive texture. After all, it is the tangible reward for earnest efforts, and many who like it view it in an almost romantic, sometimes fetishistic light. It can be a powerful aphrodisiac, too—the substance itself or simply the concept of a man coming in your mouth can be a powerful turn-on. I've illustrated the similarities come has to several different foods, but in truth there is really nothing like it. It is the genuine article; salty or sweet, thick or thin, a man's come is the part of his orgasm that shares part of him with you.

Some men revel in their ejaculate and feel emotionally good about sharing it with you, or eroticize sharing it with you—it turns them on. A man might feel hurt or pangs of rejection if you display distaste or disgust, while some men don't care, and others may dislike it as well. You never know unless you ask.

For some reason, I could never swallow. I'd think that I should, especially when I was in my last long-term relationship, because you're "supposed" to do that for someone you love.

As an earnest apprentice to the arts of fellatio, take your time getting used to everything that accompanies ejaculation, including the final result, the come itself. Take it in stages: the moment of orgasm, the contractions, and the come will become more comfortable to you as you experience them, at your own pace. When you want to find out if you like come in your mouth, or if you want to try to like it, start by first tasting it from another body part. Have him come in your hand or on another body part, then discreetly taste a little on your fingertips. This way you can try it before ending up with a mouthful of something you may not like, and you can sample it in a way that will spare his feelings if you don't like it. You can repeat this method until you gradually become more comfortable with the taste, smell, and texture. As you become more comfortable, you can aim him onto your lips or tongue. Eroticize the process— don't forget you're doing this because it's hot for both of you. Experiment with your own arousal levels as you test out your comfort; you can masturbate or fantasize to turn yourself on. Watching porn might feed the fires of fantasy and fellatio with facial or oral ejaculation. See chapter 12, "Independent Study, " for recommendations.

Close Shave

by Alison Tyler

The thing is, he shouldn't have teased me.

"Little kitty's getting furry," Tom said, warm fingers wandering down under the leopard-print sheets to find my usually well-pruned pussy. It had been a long week, and I'd skipped my routine waxing appointment in favor of a much-needed nap. But it wasn't as if I'd grown a beard. I was just a little fuzzier between my thighs than normal.

"I guess the honeymoon's over," he continued, feigning sadness.

That's when I snapped. "You're pretty furry, too," I told him, reaching down to firmly twine my own fingers in his short, blonde curls. "Maybe you should consider a visit to Darlene."

"And Darlene is—?"

"My waxer. She does men, too, you know."

"Bet she does," Tom smiled. "I'll bet she does lots of men."

"I'm serious," I told him. "Half her clients are male."

He pushed up on one arm to look at me, stunned by the thought. "They wax their pubic hair?"

Yes, I honestly know that most of the men who go to Darlene want their back hair removed, or their chests to be as smooth as a Versace boy-toy model, but I took advantage of Tom's naïveté. As I said, he'd been teasing me. "Uh, huh," I told him, nodding animatedly to show how truthful I was being. "Maybe you should try it."

"Hot wax down there? I don't think so."

"She uses cold wax, too," I continued, "and there are other methods of hair removal, you know."

"So, what are the benefits?" he asked seriously, "aside from having a strange woman's hand in your crotch." I could feel his cock stirring right below where my fingers were still nestled in his hair. This conversation was definitely appealing to his kinky side.

"Well," I purred, "you know the feeling of fucking my pussy right after a wax job when it's totally bare…?"

"'The sphinx," he said, naming the wax job I've had that completely removes all hair. Every strand. His sky blue eyes glazed slightly at the memory.

"It'll feel like that for you. Just bare, smooth skin against mine."

His hand searched out my pussy again, fingers finding the reddish fur, and he said, "Not so smooth right now, baby."

"So let's fix it." I pushed out from under the covers and padded naked down the hall. After a moment, Tom followed me to the bathroom and leaned against the cool lip of the sink as I got out the supplies. While he watched, I slipped into our shower and turned on the water. "Come on," I urged him. "Soap up first, to get everything warm and wet. Then we'll shave—"

"We?" he asked, joining me under the hot spray.

"Tit for tat," I told him, "I shave you, you shave me."

We spent a few glorious minutes sudsing each other up all over, and then I got into the frisky fun by using my pink-hued, raspberry scented, girly-girl conditioner on his pubic hair. But before he could get too turned on by this most personal shampoo session, I killed the water.

I could tell from the look on his face that he was still undecided about our little erotic adventure, so I dried off, handed over the razor, and spread myself out on the fluffy bath mat. Immediately, Tom took charge, slapping a towel around his flat waist and working me up with the lather, fingers probing and gently pinching to hold my pussy lips still. In just a short time I was bare again. And revved up. My cunt throbbed deliciously from all the attention it had just received.

Now it was his turn. "Ready, baby?" I asked. He nodded bravely and took a stand, feet apart, weight set. First, I used a small pair of silvery scissors to trim his fur. Light golden curls rained down onto the floor. Then slowly, I spread the shaving cream all over his pubes, and Tom sighed at the sensation of icy menthol against his skin. He closed his eyes when I got near him with the blade, but I have steady hands, and I whisked away all those short, blonde curls. As I rinsed him down with a soft cloth, I made sure that he could feel my hot breath on his skin. Then I parted my lips.

"What—" he murmured. "What are you doing?"

He'd thought we would immediately fuck. I understood that he'd envisioned doing it doggie-style with me bent over the sink. This is a favorite position of ours, because we can stare into the mirror on the back of the medicine cabinet, watching our reflections. But first I wanted to reward him for being such a good sport. And, honestly, the way his cock looked without any hair framing it was a total, and unexpected, turn-on. Just this majestic tower of sex, waiting to feel my warm, wet lips around it.

I put my palms on his sturdy, muscled thighs as I brought my lips to the tip of his cock. Tom sighed and traced his fingertips through my long, curly hair as I drew the next inch of his shaft farther into my mouth. There was something so unique about this experience that I had to use one hand to touch myself between my legs as I worked him. It was as if we were the most naked we'd ever been together.

Shorn. Bare. Smooth.

Sucking all the way down, I did my best to press my lips to the skin of his body, but his cock is just too long for this trick. Still, I got the contact I craved, running my fingertips along the silky skin of his balls, sliding my fingertips back behind them to press on that powerful little trigger point.

"Angel," Tom whispered. "Don't stop."

I didn't. I kept sucking and swallowing, moving back on my heels to give myself room to simply lick his shaft. My tongue in a point, I danced it up and down, caressing him, taunting him, until he couldn't handle it any longer and had to come, shooting hard down my throat so that I swallowed every drop.

We're going to keep up the bare-naked look for a while.

But I think Darlene has just lost herself a customer.

6

Before You Go Down

When it comes to erotic hot spots on the human body, nothing beats our most visual and versatile sex organ, the mouth. With this area controlled by hundreds of muscles, we can communicate intentions, ideas, and desires, and we can release streams of unrelenting dirty talk, if we choose. We can ask our lovers for what we need to get us off, or with moans and hot breaths can announce an imminent orgasm. Without a word, we can smile and flirt, we can warm up a room or a lover with peals of laughter, and most especially we can lick, bite, taste, smell, and literally inhale sex through our mouth. This sexy opening reminds everyone who looks at us that one sensual opening can lead to another, elsewhere on the body. Our lips suggest contours of genitalia, and a hint of wetness or the appearance of a tongue implies much more.

And as owners of these highly sensitive and tactile sensory organs, we do love to put things in our mouths. *Orally fixated* is a term you've no doubt heard in polite company in reference to smoking cigarettes, though inevitably everyone within earshot gets a little twinkle in their eyes mulling over the implications. It is true that as a culture we're orally fixated, constantly on the move to the next thing going into our mouth, and it's equally true that the right kind of oral stimulation can really turn us on. So maybe we're just a bunch of orally obsessed hedonists—so what? Soak up all the pleasure your lips, tongue, and entire mouth can afford you— use it to its erotic maximum every chance you get, and see how your sex life expands. Kiss, lick, and suck your lover's fingers, toes, mouth, penis, or vulva, or put on an erotic show using toys in your mouth and savor every minute.

Recognize your mouth for the sex organ it is: treat it accordingly, and learn the many delightful things you can do with it to your lover's entire genital area. Take good care of it and make it appear even sexier with some extra attention the next time you brush your teeth. Use your toothbrush to gently exfoliate your lips, and brush your tongue to make it look smoother and sexily pink. A healthy-looking mouth sends signals to potential partners on subtle levels. Use a good lip balm, and smile a lot—smiling when flirting is like waving a red flag before a restless bull. Smiling when you're going down on him will drive him wild.

Going down on your lover involves more than just putting a penis in your mouth. Giving a memorable blow job includes kissing, nibbling, licking, sucking, and caressing his entire genital area throughout the whole encounter, especially at the beginning.

Practice, Practice, Practice

It stands to reason that if you're going to be putting your sweetie's most sensitive organ in your mouth, you will want to do a little practicing and experimentation on your own first. The mouth is capable of delivering a wide variety of sensations, but you can't know how your own mouth feels unless you try out some techniques on yourself.

An organ of speech, digestion, and recreation, the tongue is a cleverly encased little package of muscle tissue, glands, fatty cells, and sensitive nerves. A mucous membrane, or *mucosa,* covers it, while the top surface, or *dorsum,* contains taste buds sensitive to touch and flavors, and serous glands that secrete some of the fluids in saliva. According to Paul Joannides in *The Guide to Getting It On!* we create and swallow saliva at the amazing rate of ten thousand gallons in a lifetime. Nerves leading from the tongue are stimulated by taste buds that react with chemicals in anything moist. The brain interprets these nervous impulses as sensations of feeling and taste. The total flavor of anything we put in our mouth comes from the combination of taste, smell, touch, texture or consistency, and temperature sensations. The tongue, with its thousands of nerve endings, talks of sweet chocolate pleasures, shouts pain when we bite it, and quietly whispers messages of erotic impulse to our big brain, all on its own.

Our lips and mouth are controlled by hundreds of muscles, always in motion, seemingly never at rest as we laugh, smile, frown, unconsciously clench our jaw, or suck on our tongue. This busy network of muscular filigree allows us to slacken our jaw, wiggle or undulate our tongue, or make the insides of the mouth into a means of suction that can draw a milkshake through a straw or give a penis pleasure. The strokes, licks, and combinations of suction that you'll want to incorporate into your oral arsenal are best first tried on you—or rather, your fingers.

First, wash your hands. Then, using the sensitive hollow of your palm, see how your lips feel grazing, nuzzling, and kissing your hand. Don't worry about how you look; just concentrate on how it feels, because it is similar to how your lover will feel when you do the same to him. Press your flattened tongue against your palm, and vary the pressure. Give your hand a long, slow lick, and repeat with several licks in different combinations: flat tongue, pointy tongue, soft tongue, flickers, caresses, firm strokes, writing your name. These strokes and licks can be repeated on the shaft of his cock, his testicles, and his anus and perineum. You'll notice your tongue dry out, then magically rewet itself, and you may find yourself making a lot of spit. This is what will happen when you go down on him, and the extra saliva serves as a helpful and desirable lubricant during head.

Hold your index and middle finger together, and holding them stiffly, caress the opening of your lips with your fingertips, as if your fingertips were the tip of your lover's penis. Slip them in slowly, feeling the wetness and heat of your own mouth. Next, try holding your mouth open with your tongue flattened inside, and gently thrust your fingers along the top of your tongue. It feels amazingly smooth and warm, and this is what he's going to feel. Squeeze your lips shut around your fingers, and experiment with suction. Move your fingers in and out, and feel your tongue move around on them, testing the way the tip, middle, and edges of your tongue feel. Increase and decrease the suction. Contract your throat muscles, and see how that feels. Hum, and see how it vibrates your fingers. Men like to have their penises licked and sucked to varying degrees, so it's good for you to know the difference between a little and a lot of suction. If you have a willing partner, you can find out how much he likes by having him suck your fingers the way he might want his penis sucked, and you can reproduce the suction to his satisfaction on his fingers to get it at the level he likes—and to make him really aroused in the process.

Experimenting with the way your mouth feels is important, but equally important in learning to give great head is setting aside some time to practice on your own. Practice oral sex on your own? Why, of course! You can get two of your own fingers in your mouth with ease, but penises are a whole different size and shape, and you don't have control over their firmness. Practice wrapping your mouth around a dildo, a penis-shaped sex toy, or a vegetable such as a peeled carrot, cucumber, or zucchini— do not attempt to "deep throat" any of these items, however, as a vegetable or slender sex toy could get lodged in your throat. (A dildo with a wide base would be

> *The head of my cock was so sensitive that I gasped as her tongue ring and lip ring ran over it.*

Do you have a pierced tongue? If so, you'll want to use your piercing to perform sensation experiments in the hollow of your hand. Moisten the most sensitive part of your palm, and see how it feels when you use your piercing to rub, massage, press, or tickle your hand. Familiarize yourself with pressure and sensation variations to get an idea of what your partner might feel when you run the piercing over the head or along the underside of his cock. When with a new partner, experiment slowly and gently at first, and plot your actions by his responses. If he doesn't seem to like it, stop—but I encourage you to ask him what he thinks whenever possible, because there's guessing... and then there's knowing.

fine, of course, since the base would prevent the entire toy from slipping into your mouth.) When you shop for the lucky nonhuman subject for your experimentations, be sure to select something as close as possible to the size of the penis belonging to your intended human subject. It's fine to practice on bigger ones later, but if you're just starting out, you'll want to begin with a comfortable size, or at least something close to the size of the penis you'll be going down on.

When you find a "stunt cock" you feel comfortable with, practice on it the way you would on a penis. If you're going to be giving head to a strap-on dildo, getting a copy of the one your lover will be wearing will help you practice your technique. Either way, experimenting with the feel of a penis-shaped object in your mouth will help you get used to having something of that size and girth filling your oral cavity. And if gagging is a major concern of yours, you can see what your comfort threshold is, or play around by pushing it and learning to tame your gag reflex. Read more on the gag reflex in chapter 7, "Giving Head." The more orally adventurous might want to try masturbating while practicing giving head—for a number of reasons. Becoming aroused when you practice will eroticize the act of fellatio, which can facilitate the incorporation of a new erotic behavior into your routine, especially if you feel reluctant. Also, as we become aroused and more turned on, our gag reflex lessens, and that can be interesting to experiment with. And finally, if you plan on masturbating or having an orgasm while going down, you can play around with your levels of concentration, varying your focus between yourself and your (potential) partner. But honestly, good luck staying focused on the dildo in your mouth when you come—though it can be fun trying.

Relaxation and Arousal

*My boyfriend never liked getting head before,
but now he does. He loves how I look at him
when I do it, and he goes crazy when I act like
I can't get enough of sucking his cock—which
is true.*

Whether you're about to give a hot and nasty, on-the-fly
blow job or are going to slowly and sweetly make love
to his cock, you'll really heat things up if you get him
into as heightened a state of arousal as you can. Simply
taking his penis and stuffing it in your mouth is fine if
you know your partner likes this, but in most cases this
approach will make the fellatio session a forgettable
one and will leave your partner disappointed—or it
may make him feel like you just wanted to get it over
with, which hurts. You may feel like you're erotically tor-
turing him by prolonging his pleasure with some
delicious foreplay, but the more thought, effort, and
attention you put into arousing him, the more he'll love
how you give head.

Spend time kissing and nibbling all over his body,
avoiding his genital area at first, tracing from head to toe
with your mouth and your hands. Get him used to the
way your hands, mouth, and body touch him, while you
become accustomed to the way he feels and responds
to you. Gently discover which parts he likes having
licked, and which to leave out. He might really love it
when you lick his neck but dislike it when you lick his
thighs. Lick everywhere: hands, the hollow of his
elbows, the nape of his neck. Caress his chest and kiss
his nipples. Try licking them as you might lick the sensitive underside of his cock head.

Using Your Hands

She did the one thing I enjoy the most when a woman gives me head. She grabbed the base with one hand, grabbed the middle with the other, and then sucked the head while stroking the rest of it with both hands...

Throughout the entire blow job, use your hands as much as you can to increase his arousal and comfort, and to prolong the sexual tension. Touching other parts of his body such as his chest, squeezing his nipples, grasping his hips, holding his buttocks, and stroking his thighs and stomach are highly recommended for building arousal—and may help a nervous lover relax. Many men enjoy the following techniques:

- Insert a finger in his mouth for him to suck and lick.
- Run your fingers through his pubic hair.
- Gently pull his pubic hair.
- Try lightly tugging on his testicles—some men like having them pulled or squeezed, though you should never tap or spank them (unless you have agreed to this type of sensation play beforehand).
- Push or pull up the mons (the fleshy mound over the pubic bone) to heighten erotic intensity; try rubbing it in a circular motion.
- When he is aroused, squeeze or pinch his nipples; as arousal increases, he may ask for stronger stimulation.
- Caress his buttocks, the cleft between his cheeks, or his anus. This is an oft-neglected part of his body, and he might really cherish your attention to the area.

Male Genital Massage

Now, this is the part that drove me crazy: she would put her ring finger and thumb together to make a ring and lightly stroke from the top of the head down to the midway point while caressing my balls with the other hand. I almost went ballistic.

Giving his entire genital area a sensual massage, or even employing just a few erotic massage techniques, can heighten any oral encounter. Whether you're looking to add to a lengthy lovemaking session or want to knead and rub him into a frenzy before you go down on him, male genital massage will help you meet your desired goal. Genital massage, like a regular massage, is a very sensual form of contact and is very relaxing for the recipient. You can use erotic massage techniques during a full-body massage, to give him an appetizer before the main course of oral sex, or simply employ the strokes and combinations to give him a mind-blowing hand job.

You can give a dry massage, but using a lubricant is highly recommended. Oils are fine to use if you're just giving him a hand job, but they aren't recommended if you're going to be putting him in your mouth or vagina, or are going to be using latex barriers such as condoms later. Oil will coat your mouth and will take a long time to clear, it wreaks havoc on the delicate pH in the vagina (and is difficult to flush out), and nothing breaks a condom like a little oil. If you do use oil, stay away from heavily scented products that might irritate his urethral opening or cause an allergic reaction: use sweet almond or olive. Water-based lubricants sold specifically for sex are best to use, especially if you want to keep your options open. If you know you're going to transition from a genital massage to a blow job, select a lubricant that tastes okay—but know that you won't find one that tastes great. For information on flavored lubricants, see chapter 4, "Know the Hard Facts: Health Considerations."

When you take a moment to marvel at what can be done with a pair of hands, it's easy to see what sensual tools they are. They can render touches that send shivers up spines, and with literally thousands of nerve endings, they *feel*, and transmit pleasure to us, their owners. Don't be surprised if giving your male partner an erotic massage turns you on.

Make sure your hands are warm and the skin feels soft. Before you begin, take time out to make sure your fingernails are trimmed and smooth and you don't have any rough spots. Remove rings and bracelets, or anything else that might get in the way or snag.

You can massage his cock in any number of places or positions, such as seated on the couch or standing in the shower, but you'll have an easier time and better access if he's lying down. Whether he's lying on a massage table draped with towels or doing dishes at the sink, start with light touches and strokes all over his torso and abdomen, upper thighs, and hips. Cup your hand over his genitals and hold it still for a moment. Press lightly, and begin to knead your hand in a barely discernable squeezing motion. Press his cock against him with the flat of your hand, and push it from side to side. You can gently cup his balls, and you can also rub his mons with flattened fingers, where his penis meets his body (you might want to review chapter 2, "The Anatomy of a Man's Pleasure"). Next, warm the lubricant between your hands (remember, there is no such thing as too much lubricant) and move on to these massage techniques:

- Press the palm of your hand on the shaft his penis and slowly squeeze repeatedly, staying in one place on the shaft. Try this at the base, in the middle, at the top.
- Try stroking with fingertips only. Stroke, pull, knead, or tap them lightly up and down along the entire shaft.
- Grasp his cock and pull it downward, and use your other hand to press on his mons. You can hold his cock in place and rub the mons in a circular motion.
- Circle your hand around the base, and pull it to the end in one long, continuous stroke.
- Reverse the stroke, starting at the head and going from tip to base.
- Try the long stroke from the base, and add a gentle twist when you reach the head. This might be too intense for some men (the head is sensitive to stimulation), but others will love it. Experiment to see if he likes the twist at the head only, or along the shaft.
- Using one hand, begin one long stroke from the base, and when you reach the head, use your other hand to follow behind the first in another stroke.
- With fingers circled around the shaft, knead and pull.
- Add your other hand to cup, fondle, or gently tug on his testicles.
- You can apply strokes with his penis pointed up, down, or in the direction of either of his hips. Many men enjoy having their penis pulled downward and back, toward their butt, but some guys will find this uncomfortable. When in doubt, ask.
- Using two hands, clasp your fingers and wrap your hands around his cock. Stroke up, down, or up and down. You can twist your hands right and left.
- With clasped hands, hold his cock still and massage in little circles with your thumbs all over the shaft and head.

- Use the index fingers and thumbs of both hands to make firm rings around him. Stroke, pull, twist.
- Cup your hand over just the head, with your fingers extended down the shaft; twist back and forth as if to juice a lemon.
- Use two hands together, pressed flat against one another with his penis in between. Gently rub your hands together, or squeeze them together for up and down strokes.
- Experiment with cupping and tugging on his balls as you use one-handed strokes.
- Try strokes that begin at his balls and continue past the head of his penis.
- Good, old-fashioned up-and-down with one hand (or two) is always a winner. Vary the pressure and rhythm.
- Hold his penis at the base in one hand, and put the shaft between your index and middle fingers, giving a slight pinch as you stroke.
- Place one hand at the base and one at the top. Twist in opposite directions.
- On his perineum, gently stroke, knead, or rub in circles.
- Some men will love the addition of anal stimulation to a massage. You can massage just at the outside of his anal opening, or add penetration. See chapter 10, "More Techniques," for details on anal play.
- Alternate any of these techniques with the open-hand massage you started with.
- If you choose to do a dry massage, you can add a twist by placing a soft fabric (like silk) between your hands and his cock. Dry massage is fun on uncircumcised men, because you can add pulling or rolling around of the foreskin. Be careful not to jerk too hard on the foreskin at the head of his cock when you use firm, pulling strokes.

Gauging His Response

When you're massaging, nibbling or licking your guy, it's easy to oversimplify his response to the pleasure you're giving: erect cock equals good, soft cock equals bad. But that's only part of the story, if it's a part at all—not all men respond to intense pleasure and satisfaction with a hard-on. Guys who get erect and stay erect throughout the duration of a blow job or an erotic massage are still experiencing a range of reactions to different ways they're being touched. Men whose penises fluctuate from hard to soft, or are mostly soft for the duration, will be feeling similarly, enjoying certain things you are doing more than others. But how do you know what he's responding to, and what it means? Asking him what's going on is ideal, though not always practical, or even possible.

> *She had her eyes on me the whole time. She went all the way to my balls, then came back slowly...*

There will be times when all you have to go by is his body language, perhaps accompanied by moans, groans, sharp intakes of breath, and possibly some cute yummy noises. Learning to take cues from his body language is essential, especially when things begin to heat up. As he becomes more aroused, you'll notice tension in his jaw or neck muscles, or he might tense the muscles in his thighs, curl his toes, or clench his fists. Ideally, he'll let you know if he wants more of anything by telling you, but he may just move his pelvis: closer, away from you, right or left. He might reposition your hands or mouth. Some men might pull your head down with their hands, grinding upward into your face, grabbing your ears or hair—this might be hot for you or really not okay at all. If you don't like having your head guided or touched, let him know before you get started that this activity is off the menu. But if it happens and you don't like it, simply move his hands firmly to your shoulders or onto his own hips.

On one end of the response scale, some men are loud, vociferous, openly appreciative lovers who let you know how they feel about every stroke, while others are quiet and withdrawn as they savor the pleasure. Chances are he's somewhere in the middle of the scale, but sometimes it's hard to tell if he really likes the way you're twisting your hand around the head, or if the pace of your strokes is fast or slow enough. When in doubt, try to have him show you what he likes; take his hand and gently place it where you're unsure.

When incredible, roller-coaster-ride, death-defying sex occurs between two people, it's because each know what the other wants. In sex, communication is crucial, and though it seems like a simple act, fellatio is no exception. Since every man is unique anatomically, all men respond to pleasurable touch differently. One man may like having his penis grabbed roughly, while another may only like it touched gently until he's on the brink of orgasm. One man might like the intense suction that a mouth can provide, while another will love the way your mouth feels wrapped lightly around him, moving slowly. Also, different parts of his penis will like to be touched more than others—many men report having a "sweet spot," though this spot can be in different places on different guys. Some men won't have a favorite spot, or it might be in different places depending on the type of erotic play you're sharing, his mood, or even the environment you're in. Ask him what he likes, and chances are he'll tell you.

Learn the anatomy of his penis and what places are sensitive to stimulation. Generally, the head, the underside of the head, and the ridge running along the underside of the penis are the more sensitive areas, but you should find out if he has a preference for where he likes to be touched—and when he likes to be touched there. For instance, the opening to his urethra (the piss slit) may be too sensitive to touch when you begin fellating him, but as he gets close to orgasm, flicking it with your tongue could drive him wild. Some men may love having their balls gently tugged during fellatio, but only at the beginning, middle, or end of the session. To really find out what he likes, you're going to need to ask specific questions. If you ask him if it feels good, he'll most likely say "yes" no matter what you're doing, and that's not enough information to go on. Here are some suggestions for questions:

- Do you like it (gripped, squeezed, tugged, stroked, licked) like this?
- Do you like being touched here? Ask this as you touch a spot with your tongue. Then touch another, and ask if he likes it more than the first. Then another…Stop and linger where he really likes it, and note that spot for later.
- Do you want it stroked harder? Softer?
- Do you want me to go faster? Slow down?
- Do you want it sucked harder? Softer?
- What else would you like me to do while I do this?

Foreplay Games for Lovers

A playful—and often very arousing—game that works on any body part is the One to Ten game. This delightful game is actually a sneaky strategy to determine his desired levels of stimulation, and it can be used throughout your lovemaking session. Because your lover's excitement levels change throughout the sexual response cycle, this game can be a helpful tool with a noncommunicative partner when you're trying to figure out what he likes. Here's how to play:

Tell him that you want to hear a number between one and ten when you touch him. The number one means he wants the lightest possible touch, and a higher number turns up the volume, ten being the top of the scale. When you begin touching or licking, you'll probably be at one, and as his arousal increases, so will the volume—and his arousal may go up and down, so pay attention. Try this out on any appealing erogenous zone: neck, nipples, the tip of his penis, testicles, perineum, or anus.

Of course, you can turn the tables with this game to conduct additional "research." Have him lick, kiss, nibble, and suck on various parts of your body, telling you what one is to him, and you can find out what a ten really means to him. This may require hours of research and a number of experiments to determine the precise levels of application.

Lovers in the beginning stages of foreplay can play a fun game that's basically an adult version of the children's game Red Light, Green Light. This game helps you determine where his erogenous zones are and can be used with any type of touch: fingers, lips (kisses), tongue (licks), face (nuzzling), or if you're daring, a sex toy or penis. To play this game, tell him that you're going to touch him in different places all over his body (and be sure to tell him with what) and that you want him to tell you one of three colors in response; red, green, or yellow. Red means "No, don't touch there"; yellow is neutral (but doesn't mean "Stop"); and green is "Yes! Right there!" Take note of what he likes and when, and you'll gradually become an unforgettably attentive, and incredibly desirable, lover.

You might want to try playing a little game called Sweet Surprise that pushes the boundaries of playfulness, trust, and power. First, assemble a variety of items that produce various physical sensations: pieces of silk, velvet, fur, rubber, or leather; ice and a cup of hot tea; a feather (or feathers); a vibrator; and if you already play with sensation a little, a small whip, a slapper, or some clips. Finally, a blindfold, and you.

Tell him that he is going to be the blindfolded subject of a sensation experiment. You can choose to allow him to see the assembled items beforehand, or not. You also have the option of restraining his wrists and ankles, if he agrees that this will enhance the game. Then, once he is blindfolded and his clothes are removed, begin touching him with different things, going slowly, using one item at a time. Ask him to identify the sensations as you go along—having him describe them to you will give you clues about how he's responding. Alternate between touching him with a piece of fake fur or velvet, and your mouth. Work your way all over his body, saving his penis and testicles for last. Gradually increase the number of kisses and strokes you give him as you incorporate his cock into the mix. Use the ice and hot tea to warm and cool your mouth alternately, if you wish. Tell him to keep describing the way your mouth feels when you are going down on him. For more about blindfolds and how to use them, see chapter 10, "More Techniques."

Don't Stop

by Alison Tyler

She's got the strap-on in place, and she comes toward the bed in a blur. I see pale skin. Sleek leather harness. Hard, pink cock. Then my vision vanishes as the black velvet blindfold covers my eyes and she easily fastens the Velcro at the back of my head. Ariel's always quick at these moments, her fingers moving with speed and finesse. There's never a false motion, never a wasted gesture.

"Suck it, Davey," she says now, but the words aren't necessary. My lips are already parted, meeting her toy and bathing the length with the heat and wetness of my mouth. I run my tongue over the ridges, meant to represent veins, the rippling bulges, the bulbous head. The taste is oddly erotic, yet totally unreal, as I'm sucking plastic instead of skin. But the erotic movements, those powerful thrusts that seal her body to me, are all her. Sex in motion. At some point, the cock will become her, as well, and I'll lose my recognition of where Ariel stops and the tool begins.

"Harder," she says, but I'm already there, fiercely working my mouth along the length, drawing her in deep. I know how to do this, although I've never gone down on another man, never even come close. Instinctively, I just know how to suck cock. Probably because I like to have mine sucked.

I try hard to swallow her toy down to the root, and she groans the way I would in a switched position, and then murmurs encouraging nonsense phrases to me. Words that have no meaning at all, but keep me going in the same direction. Her hands stroke through my short black hair. Her fingertips cradle my face, skim my evening shadow, trace over the bones beneath the skin. She is rough and gentle at the same time, and I need it just like that.

"Don't stop—"

Fuck, is it good. As I lie on my back on the bed, my lithe baby positioned on my chest, the smell of her cunt reaches me easily. I know she's getting wetter under that harness, can actually feel the liquid of her arousal spreading down the split of her thighs to my upper body. Rich and sweet, the scent makes me yearn to taste her, but it makes me sad as well because it means that soon—too soon—we will have to move onto something else. Another phase of the evening's entertainment.

When Ariel reaches a certain simmering point, she is simply unable to wait. The tool will come off and her pretty pussy will be pressed to my face so that I can fully please her. Or she'll move so that we can 69, releasing my wrists from the cold metal cuffs so that I can touch her naked cunt, stroke her ripe ass, slide my fingers into her holes. Or she'll make me roll over and the cock will find its slippery wet way between my ass cheeks. Wet from my own mouth, that tool will thrust hard. Thrust home.

But right now, I'm allowed to swim in the pure pleasure of suckling. And I relish it. Closing my eyes, I do all the magic tricks I know to make her feel the way I feel when she goes down on me. Because, oh, does Ariel know some tricks. Right there in the forefront of my mind is the image of her between my legs, her hungry mouth busy. So busy.

Ariel is a master of blow jobs. She makes it seem as if she actually breathes my skin, no longer needing air. There are no hesitations when she sucks cock. Just long, smooth strokes of her mouth on my rod, her tongue milking me, adding pressure, creating soft, soothing sensations. I mimic each of these motions, trying my best to emulate her power, her posture. Trying my best to become her. As in this little game that we play she has become me.

I give it every thing I've got. My tongue flicks along the length, making swirls, drawing lines. Then I just suck on it, feeling my cheeks indent as I work hard to please a plastic cock. And when she says the words I love to hear, I obey them without a thought.

"Don't stop, Davey. Don't stop. Don't stop."

Giving Head

Fellatio is a composition performed in three easy pieces. You conjure and build arousal with playful and purposeful oral foreplay, then you increase pleasure and establish a rhythm with specific techniques, and in the final crescendo, your rhythm combines with your mouth and hands to bring him to an orgasmic peak. These are the three main components in the art of giving mind-blowing head. Once you learn the steps and techniques, you will develop your own personal style. Pay close attention to the way the action is layered, and you'll most certainly get explosive results that will have you both grinning from ear to ear.

Your First Tastes

She lay her head on my stomach and licked, nibbled, and sucked me for what seemed hours.

Taking the time to savor his smell and taste and feel everything to the fullest in the initial stages of fellatio is similar to enjoying an appetizer before the main course. Rushing to paradise can be fun sometimes, but going slowly prolongs his pleasure and makes for a much more memorable experience. Wanting to dive right in, or rather, plunge it in, is a delicious urge. When the passion and desire is at the point that you can't get into each other's clothes fast enough, then the eye-popping sensation of his cock going straight into your hot little mouth is fitting. Although, when he's that hot and bothered, why not make him want it even more by slowing down the action?

If you're putting him in your mouth for the first time, or are nervous about the whole process, then let time be on your side as you get acquainted with the look, aroma, and flavor of his genitals. As you transition from foreplay to fellatio, gradually narrow your attentions to his groin area, and spend extra time touching and kissing the area around the pubic region. If you've been giving him an erotic massage, then you're already familiar with the sensory information that comes with being near him. As you kiss and nibble closer to his cock and balls, take a moment for you both to adjust to the feeling of having your face near his genitals. If he's wearing underwear, you can kiss or even mouth his cock and balls through the fabric—this feels amazing to the recipient. Should you want to take his underwear off, slowly slide down one side at a time as you kiss and nuzzle his hips and the curve of his lower abdomen and hips.

When you begin to incorporate his penis and testicles into your attentions, start out with light kisses that are all soft lips and no tongue. Combine your kisses with other types of touch elsewhere, such as caresses and light squeezes with your hands; you can also press your face against his genitals to fully incorporate the action. Some men will be delighted if you run their penis over your face and neck, especially if it's done with a sweetly salacious smile. The extra contact when you're going down on him makes a big difference between "any old blow job" and getting head from someone who really wants him to feel good. Add long, languorous licks where his inner thighs meet his torso. Light, hot, focused breath on different parts of him provides a nice teasing touch.

If you're feeling unsure about taking the first taste, run your closed lips over the shaft of his penis and the head. Inhale, moisten your lips, and try giving the skin an open-mouthed kiss, sans tongue. Taste your lips. He might be one of those juicy guys who produces a liquid called pre-come when aroused, and you may want to sample that flavor before you put him in your mouth. This is an activity for "fluid bonded" couples; read more about it in chapter 4, "Know the Hard Facts: Health Considerations." Pre-come tastes slightly different from ejaculate; the flavor is generally light, but it differs from man to man. With a thoughtfully placed stroke, you can pick up a little pre-come on your fingertips and discreetly sample the way it tastes. If you don't like it, you can use the opportunity of not yet having started fellatio to transition to another activity you feel more comfortable with.

Now you can invite your tongue to the party, if you haven't already. While giving his crotch every other type of attention, you can gradually incorporate little licks or tongue flickers to his penis head, shaft, and base, his testicles, and where his scrotum meets his body, and you can lift his balls and lick his perineum. Use your hand to guide his penis into positions that make it easy for you to reach every spot, especially the sweet spots he responds to positively. He might really like being licked along the underside of the shaft, though he may prefer a spot at the base, up the center, at his circumcision scar (if he's circumcised), or on the underside of the head. He may also like it all around the lower ridge of the head, where it mushrooms off the shaft, or at a particular point along that ridge. Some men really enjoy having their urethral opening (where urine leaves the penis, also called a "piss slit") tongued and licked, though not all guys like this; you'll have to pay attention to his reaction.

> Stay hydrated! It's no fun to go down on someone when you have a dry mouth, and giving head can be thirsty work. If you've been drinking alcohol, you're going to get dehydrated faster than nondrinkers, but either way it's a good idea to keep a glass of water nearby (if you can) to keep your kisser moist.

This is a terrific time to experiment and play with different tongue techniques. Again, it is highly recommended that you use your hands to guide his penis, adding the extra pleasure of fondling or lightly squeezing his balls. With your tongue, you can do the following:

- Flicker sensitive spots, such as those mentioned above. Flicker side to side or up and down, or give light taps.
- Press your tongue flat on the head.
- Point your tongue and give pressing strokes anywhere.
- Soften your tongue and slide sloppy trails everywhere.
- Give long, slow licks, as you would to an ice cream cone.
- Speed up the long licks, then slow them again.
- Hold your tongue stationary and run the head of his cock over it.
- Lightly lick his balls, or slather them with saliva.

- Gently suck one or both of his balls into your mouth. The popular term for this is tea bagging.
- Incorporate your soft lips (no teeth), and run your lips and tongue up and down the shaft, or over the head. Add a little suction if you like.
- If he's uncircumcised, pull the foreskin back with your fingertips to kiss and lick him. You can also leave the foreskin in place and sweep your tongue around inside—but go easier than you would with a circumcised man, because uncut penises are usually more sensitive to stimulation on the head.

Watch his reactions to your focused licking and flicking. If he seems to be pulling away, then that spot might be too sensitive to what you're doing: back off and move on to another area, or change your tongue technique to something less intense. But if he's getting really hard, if his hips are beginning to thrust, you've got him right where you want him.

The Pierced Penis

A penis piercing can change the way you use your mouth and hands, and you'll want to take into account the possible differences in sensation for him. First, keep in mind that piercings are susceptible to infection throughout the healing period, so you'll want to avoid oral sex until he's done healing (two weeks is a safe waiting period), especially if you practice safer sex— your saliva can inhibit his healing, and you'll be sharing bodily fluids, because genital piercings can bleed during the first twenty-four to forty-eight hours; beyond that, piercings can bleed for about a week during erections. Once the site is healed, a piercing is perfectly clean, just the same as a pierced ear. A piercing will make his penis more sensitive to stimulation, especially the specific area that's pierced.

There are several different styles of piercings and jewelry that can adorn them, including steel or gold hoops

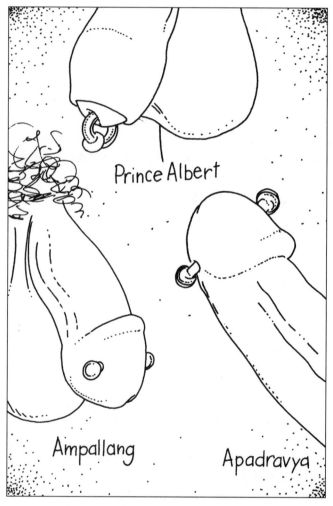

Illustration 7. Genital Piercings

or barbells. A Prince Albert piercing passes through the eye (urethral opening) and either downward through the head's underside (most common), or upward through the head's top (a "reverse"). Ampallangs pass horizontally through the glans and not through the urethra; several can be worn at a time. The Apadravya passes through the head's ridge and can also be worn in sets. Experiment to see what types of sensation he likes on his piercings, if he likes any specific attention on them at all. Some men might like them flicked lightly with your tongue, gently tugged by lip suction—but some won't want attention focused on the piercing at all, preferring to let the piercing add to the typical range of sensations in a blow job. Should a piercing come out in a heated moment, don't panic—this can happen, and it doesn't hurt. Just let him know it came out and ask him what he wants to do.

Using Your Mouth and Hands

When she was done teasing me, she leaned down, raised my cock slightly with the hand that had been teasing my balls, and took what felt like my whole cock in her mouth. No licking, no teasing, just one long slide into her hot, wet mouth. It was an incredibly erotic experience, partly because I was so horny, partly because of the contrast between her mouth and the cold air, and partly because it was so smooth and simple.

When you're ready to put him in your mouth—and he's *really* ready to be in your mouth—you have a few choices about how you want to switch your oral ministrations into higher gear. Either way, when his penis first makes contact with the heat and wetness that's inside your mouth, he's going to feel like he's gone straight to heaven. Don't be surprised if you get an appreciative gasp or moan.

Before you wrap your lips around his delicate member, know that the one major rule about blow jobs is to keep your teeth off the playing field at all times. It's pretty easy to avoid having him hit your molars, but your front teeth (or any rough dental work) can turn an oral outing into a trip he'll never want to take with you again. Even lightly and imperceptibly, teeth can scrape the thin and sensitive skin of the penis. Cover your front teeth by wrapping your lips over them. You can minimize any discomfort you may feel on the inside of your mouth by keeping your lips slightly tensed or pursed. It's also good for comfort (and to vary the stimulation he's getting) to keep your lips on the move. Vary the way you pucker, purse, and wrap your lips as you move him in and out of your mouth and alternate your sucking and kissing. A few men will like the sensation of light nibbling with your teeth or feeling them run feathery-light on their cock— but this is an activity that should be talked about before you try it. Many men will get nervous in all the wrong ways if you rub them with your teeth and they don't want it.

Needless to say, when you begin to put his penis in your mouth, you aren't going to begin ramming up and down, as fast as you can—take it slowly. Put him in, then back out, and repeat the process as an intermediate stage of oral foreplay. How you play around with this initial in and out is up to you. When his penis starts making the first dips into your mouth, try choosing among these suggestions:

- You can gradually work in the sensation of going into your mouth, alternating sliding the head just between your lips, and other licks and kisses you're already doing.
- You can stick your flattened tongue out, hold it perfectly still, and slide him slowly in, then wrap your lips around and apply a little suction.
- Run the tip of the head around your moistened lips (as if it were lipstick), pausing to push him in, around, back in, repeat...
- You can, of course, shove him in suddenly. This works well if you hold still for a few moments after shoving to let the sensation sink in.
- Begin pulling him in with your lips, moving forward and back, but go farther down with each forward motion.
- Try wrapping your hands around his hips or buttocks, with the tip of his cock held in place with your lips. Pull him in and out with these "handles."

If I gag, I just jack him off for a minute.

At this stage, you'll be liberally using your hands not only to maintain sensual contact with your partner but also to keep the stimulation going on his penis as your mouth leaves and returns. One or both hands will hold him steady as you put him in and out of your mouth. You can also rely on your hands to stroke him and duplicate your mouth's movements if your jaw needs a rest. Use your hands to guide his penis, and always keep both hands on him somewhere; hips, butt, stomach, thighs, balls, chest. You can lightly run your fingernails over non-ticklish areas such as his thighs or chest, tease his pubic hair, and stroke or massage the line from belly button to pubic bone. You can also reach up and caress his neck, face, and lips, and some guys love it when you slip a finger or two in their mouth to lick and suck.

The way to deal with big dicks is to use your hand as an extension to your mouth. Lots of saliva. Then keep stroking him and lick his balls. And below his balls. Back up for more sucking, then back down for more ball licking. Perhaps tickle his asshole if he likes that.

The Eyes Have It

One time I asked her to look at me, and she did so while continuing to give me head. I told her how good it felt, what an incredible turn-on it was to watch her suck my cock, and how it was even more of a turn-on to look into her eyes while she did so.

We're visual creatures by nature. Blow jobs can take this principle to delirious heights. Since the person receiving head can watch the action, why not crank up the volume by putting on a show? Eye contact is where it's at when you want to heighten the sexual tension. You can stare intensely into his eyes as you go at it, or punctuate your activities by stealing coy glances now and then.

Touching his testicles enhances what you're doing to his penis, and to the rest of him. The balls are often neglected in oral sex, even though they're a major pleasure zone. A few men will dislike having them touched at all, but most will appreciate having them included in the fun. Touch them lightly at first; if the response is positive, you can cup and hold them, give light squeezes or tugs, caress them with your fingertips, lift them slightly and hold them still, or reach behind them and massage or stroke his perineum. Prolong these initial stages of having him in your mouth for as long as you want, and remember that the longer you make it last, the more turned on he'll get.

Whenever I feel horny and want to get off, all I have to do is close my eyes and think back to that day. I can still feel her mouth around my cock and the way she never neglected my balls. It was amazing.

Strokes and Combinations

Her head was bobbing up and down, one of her hands was in my mouth, and the other one was massaging my balls! I mean, I was in ecstasy!

Some people spend years using a single blow job technique on their lovers—and there's nothing wrong with that, as long as everyone's ecstatically happy with the results. But not every sexual encounter is the same in tone or duration, and not all men respond overwhelmingly to cookie-cutter oral sex formulas. It's a good idea to mix it up, and make the blow job match the man and the mood. There are many different strokes and ways to combine them with one another and with the techniques you've already learned. Using more than one, and going slowly through a catalog of moves, lends length and body to your session, while giving your lover an outstanding oral sex experience.

The crux of your oral technique is the way you use your hand (or hands) in accompaniment with your mouth. The key to doing this is to use a hand in tandem with your mouth on his shaft, as an extension of your mouth. Wrap one hand around his cock, with your index finger and thumb meeting at the top, and keep these fingers against your lips. Moving up and down with your hand locked to your lips, you make an intensely pleasurable, tight tube for him to slide in and out of. Most men like a firm grip, but not too firm; test your grip on two of your fingers to see how it feels before you get started. If you're not sure, you can always have him put his hand on yours and show you.

> *He would take the tip of his tongue, run it along the length of it for a while, very sensually, always varying the pace but never feeling out of rhythm. He also did the one thing I enjoy the most when a man gives me head. He grabbed the base with one hand, grabbed the middle with the other, and then sucked the head while stroking the rest of it with both hands...*

Using your hands along with your mouth is an important technique, and it has several beneficial side effects. Besides making your mouth into a pleasurable space that he can slide entirely into, your hands can also enhance his pleasure by moving in different ways or adjusting constriction at any point in your up-and-down motions. And it can provide a way for you to minimize how deep he goes into your mouth, so if you're concerned about gagging or hip thrusts, you can use your hand as a buffer. If your jaw, neck, or anything else gets sore or tired, you can rest your mouth and keep the stroking and rhythm continuous, not breaking contact. In fact, you can give yourself a stealthy rest by moving back and stroking him while looking at him seductively, and he'll be none the wiser. Your hand-and-mouth motion comes into play when you "deep throat" him; read about how to do this in chapter 9, "Deep Throat."

Survey your choices when it comes to strokes and the combinations you can create with other sensations. Pick some and try them in combination to see what he likes; you'll notice that a particular way you are going down on him will turn him on more. Then begin to focus your energy on the type of stroke he responds to pleasurably, and establish a rhythm. Always keep your upper lip curled protectively over your teeth—a nip at the wrong moment is unsettling. When he starts to respond to a particular technique, you'll begin your rhythm. Establishing a rhythm is your goal, but be sure to stay with each technique you use long enough for him to get used to it. Don't rush through changing techniques, or change what you do with each stroke— this is frustrating for the recipient, who is trying to focus on arousal and orgasm. The following strokes are your road to rhythm:

- To do the master stroke, the basis for fellatio, keep your hand against your lips, and bob up and down.
- Try long strokes, short, slow strokes, or a rapid in- and-out motion.
- Adjust the pressure in your hand by making it snug for entire strokes, or constrict your grip when you go down to the base of the shaft, or at the head.
- Vary your suction. Increase it for a few strokes, then release. Try using more suction on either up or down strokes.
- Play around with the different ways you can cre- ate suction. Try pulling with your lips, by creating a vacuum with your tongue, or pulling by con- stricting your throat. Each way will feel different to him.
- Try using no suction at all, with either a tight or a loose hand.
- Hold your mouth still and pump with your hand.
- Pull the foreskin down tightly while only your mouth goes up and down.

- Twist your head as you go up and down. Try it for the length of a whole stroke, or only when you reach the tip. Twist on up or down strokes, or both.
- Twist only your hand, with the same variations.

- Hold still for a moment and squeeze only your mouth and throat in rhythm.
- Experiment with keeping your tongue in constant motion.
- Allow him to make the motion by thrusting his penis in your mouth while you hold still—this is called irrumation.

> It stands to reason that once he's very aroused and close to orgasm, he probably won't know exactly what you're doing; he'll just know if it feels good or not. It's up to you to remember what worked and what didn't.

On Gagging

Touch the back of your tongue with a toothbrush, and you'll feel that dreadfully familiar involuntary reflex shared by all—you'll gag. The entire back of the mouth and soft palate are wired with nerves that are auto-programmed to trigger muscular convulsions in your throat when touched, constricting the opening of the throat and sending signals to your stomach to begin a queasy lurch. This is how the body protects itself from choking on oversized objects. We are not serpentine; we cannot unhinge our jaws. Put something bigger than your mouth into your mouth, and you will gag.

Everyone gags at some point during a blow job. It may take several blow jobs or several years of giving them to gain control over your reflex, and even sea-soned pros at fellatio gag sometimes. At first it's unsettling and challenging. Your eyes will water, and your nose may run—some partners find this sexy. But with time, practice, and comfort with oral sex, you can learn to overcome your body's natural instinct to push back at whatever's pushing in. No one ever overcomes it completely, but there are techniques that help, and staying cool-headed is important.

> I try to deep throat, but my stomach always churns. What I do is take him really deep for one stoke, then not deep for a few, then deep again for one stroke. Guys really love this, and they don't seem to notice that it's for only one stroke that they're really deep.

Learn to make incorporate your anti-gagging techniques into your act. The Flying Wallendas were the greatest tightrope walkers in the history of circus performance. They believed that when learning tightrope, one should avoid the aid of tethers or nets, so as not to get too dependent upon them. The thinking was that if you came to rely on these aids, you would take their existence for granted and someday forget that they weren't there, and fall. This encouraged them to practice falling, to the extent that they made falling into an art form. When they fell during performances, they would slip and cling to the rope with such style and grace that everyone believed it was all part of the act. You can do the same with gagging, a potentially unsexy response to an intimate sex act: when you feel yourself beginning to gag, make pulling him out of your mouth and taking a rest until the feeling subsides part of your act. Learn techniques for overcoming your gag reflex in chapter 9, "Deep Throat."

Rhythm: The Essence of a Blow Job

As you sense his excitement building, narrow your focus onto one or a combination of two specific stroke techniques he likes. Using these, establish a beat—a consistent and predictable rhythm with the strokes. When using one stroke, go at a steady pace and try gradual increases and decreases of your tempo. With two stroke combinations, use one for five or six beats (strokes), then switch to the other stroke for the same amount of time and back again. For instance, you can bob up and down the length of his shaft using your hand pressed to your lips and a little suction, then switch to holding the head in your mouth while you stroke with your hand, then switch back.

Men differ in their rhythm preferences, and you'll find that he may require an increase, decrease, or no change at all in order to achieve orgasm. You can find out by asking if he wants it faster or slower, but don't interrupt the activity too much or you'll risk decreasing the heightened state you've got him in—keep stroking him with your hand if you pause to ask. You might ask him to masturbate for you; watching what he does right before he orgasms is extremely instructional. But these options aren't always available, and sometimes you'll just have to pay very close attention to his response. When you make a change and see his pre-orgasmic tension increase or decrease, you'll know. Some men will love a steady, firm, driving rhythm, then want a few quick strokes to make them come. Others won't require any change at all and will orgasm in one fluid movement during one of your strokes. Your rhythm (and how it's used) is what's going to make him come, so tune in to his body language (that is, if he's not disturbing the neighbors with his cries and moans of pleasure), and watch for the signs of imminent orgasm.

Bump and Grind: Pre-Orgasmic Body Language

Wanting to be the gentleman, I announced well before the fact that I was getting ready to cream. Much to my surprise and joy, she did not stop sucking...

An oncoming orgasm in a man can take many forms. He might be the vocal type, telling you he's about to come, or his moans and yummy noises could reach an audible crescendo. There are physiological signs, too. His muscles may tense in different parts of his body, such as thighs, jaw, abdomen, hands, and feet. In most men, the testicles retract, hugging the body, and the penis stiffens to its fullest point before the rhythmic contractions of orgasm begin. His hips might begin to thrust, or he might grind his pelvis in your face—sometimes quickly, in rough jerks, but sometimes the movement is subtle and barely perceptible. He could slowly seem to be getting closer and closer to your face, maybe even pushing you down a little bit—or a lot!

I love to swallow. When a guy comes in my mouth, I know he's lost control and it's so hot, I just want to drink every drop.

This is the time when a number of things can happen. He is about to ejaculate, and it's up to you where you want it to go—not only should it go where you want it, but he should come where and in whatever way turns you on. You could wait until the initial pulses and spasms begin, then pull back slightly as he comes on your tongue or lips. Or you might relish the taste and feel of him coming deep in your mouth or throat, swallowing it as he orgasms. Many people find it hot to have him come on their face, breasts, stomach, or hands, or into their open mouth, and even enjoy the association with porn's "money shots," finding that it adds to the heat of the encounter. If you hold your mouth still and close your throat, you can hold his come in your mouth and swallow it when the moment passes—or not. Pulling your head back and bringing him to orgasm with you hand is another option. Jack him off onto or into any area you want, and enjoy the show.

> *He can come on me anywhere—yum! I don't care. My tits, face, in my mouth, stomach... as long as he's coming on or in me I don't care.*

Many people enjoy it when their lover comes in their mouth, but not everyone does, and those who do like it don't always want to do it every time. When you're with a lover you're familiar with, you may recognize his body's signals that an orgasm is imminent, or you may have an agreed-upon signal. If you know you don't want him coming in your mouth and you've agreed on a signal, this is the time you'll get that signal. Then you can move him out of your mouth so he comes elsewhere. Not infrequently at this stage, men put their hands on your head, sometimes involuntarily. For many men, touching your head is affectionate; it feels good to connect with you and be fully present in the activity. Their intention may be to guide your head faster, slower, or deeper. But sometimes it feels inappropriate. If you don't like this or it makes you feel uncomfortable, you don't have to stop the session; simply move his hands to your shoulders or onto his own body. If you like the guidance or relish having him take control, then this is the right time to let go, and having his hands on your head provides the perfect way to do it.

I used to get freaked out thinking about the possibility of him putting his hands on the back of my head. But now when my boyfriend does it, it's like he just wants the contact with me, and he strokes my hair and face. It's sweet and turns me on!

When he's bucking or grinding and you know that an orgasm is right around the corner, do what you can to hang on and keep doing whatever it is you're doing. Don't stop! Hang on to his hips or buttocks if you're worried about getting bucked off, or conversely, you can control his thrusts if he's going overboard. Gripping him like this can really increase his pleasure, and some guys go crazy being held onto this way. He might also like to have his thighs immobilized before orgasm: simply hold them firmly still. Also try putting his legs together. If thrusting is unwanted, have him lie on his back for fellatio, and with your hand on his shaft you can position your forearms on his hips, using your body weight to keep his hips down. If after all the bucking and grinding is over you feel like a cowpoke with whiplash, you may want to talk about it later.

Orgasm

When he orgasms, the delightful contractions begin, and you'll feel the muscles in his cock spasm as ejaculate is released. A man can have many types of orgasms; some men can orgasm without ejaculation, when soft, or without any muscular contractions in their penises. Men with disabilities such as spinal cord injuries may experience "phantom orgasms" elsewhere in the body. Orgasms vary in length, on average anywhere from five seconds to three minutes. Some orgasms are sweat-drenched, roof-raising events; others pass with barely a sigh of released breath and a lovely glow to his cheeks—and there's everything in between.

For people who use condoms with oral sex, spitting or swallowing isn't an issue, but everyone else needs to take a minute before the act even begins to decide what they want to do. Communication is crucial no matter what you decide. If it's okay, let him know so that he can completely relax when orgasm is close—some men are acutely aware that not everyone wants to swallow and can get anxious prior to orgasm if you haven't talked about it. If it's not okay, or if you're just not sure, tell him. Most men will be glad you brought it up (and if they're not, kick them right out of bed). If you don't tell him and you try to hide an unpleasant reaction when he orgasms, you run the risk of hurting his feelings. Instead, tell him that you're not sure you want him to come in your mouth, and ask him to give you a tap on the shoulder or tell you when he is about to come.

When I suck a guy off I swallow his cum. Spitting it out is too much trouble, plus my swallowing makes him really happy.

When you want to avoid him coming in your mouth, move your mouth off of him and continue stroking his penis with your hand. He can ejaculate elsewhere:

- He can come on your closed lips.
- He can ejaculate onto other sexy places, such as your neck or chest.
- You can use both hands to stroke him to orgasm, then let one hand linger at the head and catch it when he comes.

- You can allow him to come in your mouth, but into the side of your mouth, your cheek. The ejaculate misses your tongue, where the taste buds can trigger a sensitive gag reflex. Then you can discreetly spit it into the hand on his penis.

One time he came in my mouth and I didn't think I could deal with it, but at the last minute his penis slipped into my cheek and he came there, instead of on my tongue or in my throat. It was totally different, and easier.

During orgasm you may be either pushed away from his penis, or pulled closer to maximize penis-mouth contact. He might love having you continue to stroke him all the way through his orgasm, but some men find that the head is extremely sensitive right after orgasm and can barely stand the slightest movement. Slowing your motions and stopping as he is coming is a good idea; most men will stop you if it feels too intense and they want you to hold still. You can lightly kiss and lick his cock after he comes, or you can tenderly hold it in your mouth or hand for a few minutes. Then, make your way up to eye level and see what he feels like doing next—he may just need a few minutes to relax in his post-orgasmic haze. If he's sensitive about cleanliness and scent, wipe your face with a damp washcloth (the one you thoughtfully placed by the bed earlier) before you kiss him on the face or lips.

She pulled up my underpants and pants, rezipped, buttoned, and buckled them, and lay down on my chest. We hugged and kissed, and I could smell the strong scent of my sperm from deep in her throat, and taste it on her lips and tongue.

Boys Will Be Boys
by Alison Tyler

We form a perfect union when we 69. Jarred on top and me on the bottom, cocks between lips, hands moving and roaming. The fact that he's black and I'm white simply adds to the theme. Photo negatives. Mirror images. Reflections in still water.

There are plenty of occasions when we don't take our time. Moments when it's all about the end. All about shooting, creaming, and then collapsing. During those times, the romance of our relationship fades and we just f-u-c-k—fuck. Slam into each other with everything we've got. Sweaty, groping, fists and fingers, eyes shut, mouths open.

But now, in the late-afternoon light, we are in love, and we take things slowly. I caress the sweet, swollen head of his cock using only my full lips, wet from a single lick. No tongue yet. Cradling the rounded head, teasing it with the slippery kisses that I know will make him want to go fast. He rewards—or is it tortures?—me with the same behavior. Millimeter by millimeter, he works his dreamy mouth over the tip of my throbbing dick before finally sliding his lips down the shaft.

More slowly, I suck him, paying attention to every single sensation as I pump my mouth up and down. His earthy taste, his honey smell, the way his balls hang down, the way he groans when I graze them with my fingers or tug them gently as I suck a little harder.

When I become so focused on every second, I realize that I am paying attention to more than just Jarred. More than just sex. In the still afternoon, I am aware. The mattress is firm beneath me. The sound of an old jazz record plays in the apartment next door, scritch-scratching every few bars in a way that a CD can't. The rhythm of Jarred's breathing seems to match the music. The one thing I forget about is me. I am gone, no longer important, no longer a player.

That is, until Jarred uses his teeth.

Not to bite, but to nip, so lightly that I feel I am going to cry. It's unlike any other thing he does. Unlike any other sensation I've ever experienced. He lets his lips part, lets his tongue rest behind his lower teeth, and works me up and down with just the bare edges of his teeth, the very, very tips of them. It's like being cradled between the jaws of a lion.

I see pictures in my mind when he does this. I think of Jarred at his studio, surrounded by sculptures in progress, surrounded by stone, by wet clay. I think of him with his abundant utensils and interesting tools, scratching softly in the surface. Then digging a little deeper. Making a mark.

To him, I know, I am a work in progress, a piece of art that calls out to be completed. And with his little tricks he claims me, names me, his voice a rumble behind my cock as he starts to talk.

"Suck harder," he says in a tone that is almost a whisper. "Suck me like you mean it, Michael." The rumbling vibrations of his words against my skin send me higher, and I do as he asks. My mouth closes in, the walls of my throat become tight. I am a vacuum. I am a machine. Slow becomes fast as I slide my mouth back and forth, giving him everything he wants. Who am I to hold back? Who am I to withhold pleasure?

Lips, tongue, sweet, wet mouth. Hard, soft, changing like the light changes in the room. Like the music changes one wall away. We are in tune. We are jazz. In perfect synch, we work each other. His bone moves deeper, deeper into my throat, and I swallow as forcefully as I can against him. I want to drain him. I want to devour him.

He echoes every motion. Until I forget who started what. Until I forget where I end and he begins. And then one of us does something new, and off we go on another route. My hand now around the base of his cock, holding tight there as I lick the tip. His fingers pressing up behind my balls, teasing me there, when he knows just a little pressure at that magic spot will make me want to fuck him. Roll over and just fuck him. It's like this forever. Slip-sliding up to the climax and then back down from it.

My mouth is a hungry beast, and I swallow on him once again. Jarred won't let me get away with that. He uses the whole flat of his tongue to massage and caress underneath the head of my cock, so that I release him completely and loll back on the mattress, unable to move because it feels so fucking good.

We are playing a game without rules.

Playing like boys do, to see who will win.

Any Way You Want It

Nothing is more fun than having choices and possibilities—and fellatio is amazingly adaptable to environment, preference, and personal style. You can custom-tailor a session of head to suit your needs or your partner's needs in almost any way imaginable. A position can enhance physical pleasure or a conjured fantasy. Fellatio can be the ticket to overcoming physical obstacles, such as a disability. You can use fellatio performed on a strap-on to set fire to an already sizzling sex life. Or, you can explore the ways to customize your physical approach to giving head to make it more comfortable, combat jaw fatigue, or strengthen your skills by learning how to take a penis or dildo all the way in your mouth and throat: learning to "deep throat."

Positions

Fellatio feels good to the recipient in pretty much any angle you choose to give it, and there are a lot of positions to choose from. As a sex act it affords the uniqueness

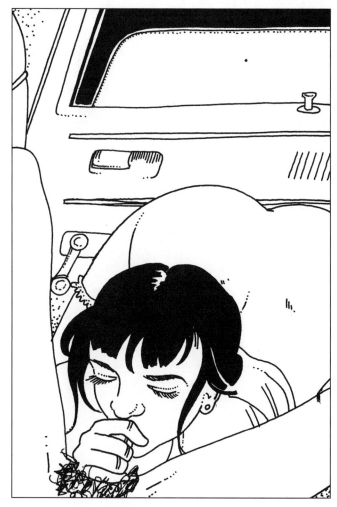

Illustration 8. Anytime, Anywhere

of being able to be performed virtually anywhere. Because it's so versatile, the positions you can use vary greatly, and they can depend on location and circumstance. Trying fellatio in new locations and new positions can spice things up; a change in your routine or simply trying something you haven't tried before can make the experience a bigger turn-on for both of you than your previous oral escapades.

Each position has advantages and disadvantages. Certain positions will afford you more access to his genitals, might make it easier for you to take more of him in your mouth, or may give you a psychological rush with their fantasy implications. However, you may find that some positions make you gag more than others because of the angle, are tough on your knees or jaw, or cause you to feel uncomfortable for other reasons. One thing to keep in mind when you consider positions is that you may be in any given position for a good amount of time, so you will want to take into account how comfortable you'll be after, say, fifteen minutes or longer. There is no established amount of time to orgasm for men, or women for that matter, and if you think that men orgasm reliably and quickly as a rule, then you're in for a surprise—and maybe some leg and neck cramps while you're at it. Choose positions that are comfy for the two of you, and don't be shy about changing positions or moving him around in different configurations.

The Consummate Position

I've always found it works best with him lying down or leaning back, and to kneel beside him approaching him perpendicularly.

The position that lends itself easily to variety and comfort is having him lie on his back with a pillow under his head on a bed, the ground, a couch, or any flat spot. It provides the best access to his entire genital area and allows him to lie back and completely relax and enjoy. This position allows you to easily include his testicles in the action, or incorporate penetration, rimming, pressure points, or any other tricks you have in store. You can place yourself between his legs, or move around his body as you like. If you're on your stomach, this position can get a little tiresome on your neck, but you can alleviate strain by changing positions, using these variations:

- On your stomach between his legs, prop yourself up on your elbows and grasp his buttocks or hips.
- With your elbows propped, have him put one or both legs over your shoulders.
- Have him hold his knees to his chest.
- Have him place his feet on your shoulders.
- Kneel or crouch between his legs, leaving your hands free to help, wander, tease.
- With his legs spread around you, keep your hands on his groin area and press his hips down using your forearms and the weight of your body on his hips.
- Wrap your arms under his thighs, and toward you over his hips. You can guide his cock easily from this position.
- Sit on his legs, forcing them flat and rendering them immobile.
- Lick from a right angle, one side or the other. You can kneel, crouch, lie sideways, or adjust pillows under you for comfort. You can face him, or face his feet.
- Sit on his chest, facing away from him. He gets a nice view, you get access to him, and the angle is good for alleviating the gag reflex.

On Your Knees, Now

My first time sucking cock was quick and nasty,
and now that's the way I like it best.

When most folks think of fellatio, the image of someone on their knees comes readily to mind. At some point in your fellatio adventures, you're bound to wind up on your knees, whether your lover is standing or seated. Kneeling might be the best possible choice for a given situation or circumstance—for instance, if you're outdoors, being spontaneous in the bathroom, shoving him up against a wall and having your way with him, or engaging in a "quickie." Your hands are free to roam, fondle testicles, guide his penis, or pull him into your mouth by his hips or buttocks. But kneeling isn't for everyone, because it is tough on the knees—though you may be having so much fun you don't notice until it's all over. If your knees ache or strain but you don't want to give up the position, switch to crouching or squatting. Crouching also makes it easier to masturbate while you fellate.

More Positions

SEATED
He can sit on the edge of a bed, chair, table, kitchen counter, car seat, staircase...anywhere. You can kneel on the floor with pillows under your knees, squat, or if he's up high enough, sit on a low chair or stool. This position is ideal for the comfort and access it provides.

SIDEWAYS
You can both lie sideways, and you can prop pillows under your head for comfort.

"SITING ON YOUR FACE."

He doesn't actually sit on your face; he puts his knees on either side of your upper torso and sits on your chest, with his penis in your face. He can also hover above your face so you can also lick his balls, suck them into your mouth, and tongue his perineum, though rimming is difficult from this angle. He can provide the thrusts, or stay still while you move your head and hands. Your hands can travel over his entire lower torso and can easily play with his ass.

THE 69 (SIMULTANEOUS RECIPROCAL ORAL SEX).

There are a couple of options for this favorite: him on top, on hands and knees over you; you on top (same thing reversed); or both of you on your sides, which may be the most comfortable of the three. Experiment with this one to see what you both like—in fact, you should experiment with all of these positions, over and over...

> *I had a girlfriend who loved to 69. She actually often forgot the up-and-down sucking motion; she got off on having her clit licked while my cock was in her mouth. She'd lie on top of me and grind her pussy against my face and just hold my erection in her mouth. I wasn't really complaining!*

> *One time he asked to 69 with me on top, and that was the best that I remember. It was such a turn-on to know he just really enjoyed having my penis in his mouth, plus I could thrust and get the sensations that I enjoyed. Sucking his dick and fucking his mouth with long, slow strokes is something I won't forget.*

What He Can Do When You're in the 69 Position
- Give you head, of course.
- Spank you.
- Penetrate you vaginally or anally with his fingers or a sex toy.
- Nothing, if he's tied up.

ON YOUR BACK

If you lie on your back, with your head tilted back off the edge of a bed or sofa, your throat is stretched and much more open than in any other position. Many people prefer this for deep throating and say it reduces the gag factor. He is standing and doing the thrusting, but you can still use your hands.

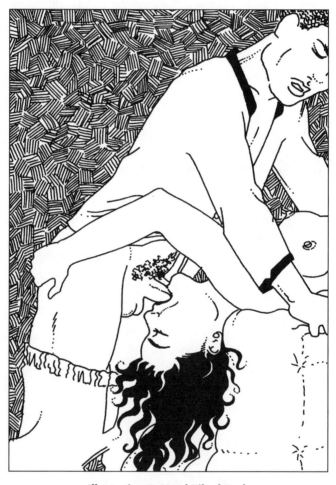

Illustration 9. Head Tilted Back

DOGGIE-STYLE

This position isn't just for penetrative sex. Lick him from behind while he's on hands and knees, pulling and sucking his penis back between his legs. Not all guys find this comfortable, but those who do will delight that you can also play with their testicles and perineum, and can fully explore rimming and anal play.

Jaw Cramp

Once you've got your stroke and rhythm going, and you're in the position of choice, you're in it for the duration. How long is that? Sorry—there's no answer to that question. It could be a few short strokes and then he explodes, or he could last longer than an all-day sucker—or he might not come at all. These scenarios are all possible, and because it takes as long as it takes, you might have a mouthful for longer than you thought. The natural, though unpleasant, side effect of it all is that your tongue may cramp, your jaw may ache, and your neck might get tired. Fellatio can put strain on jaw and neck muscles like no other sex act, which is why it's important that you start out in a comfortable position, especially if you have injuries or TMJ, or just plain get crampy muscles. The irony is, when it seems like you're just about to collapse he's usually on the verge of exploding, and no insurance company under the sun will cover your fellatio-related repetitive stress injury (RSI).

Like a distance runner, always pace yourself from the start and keep a steady, slow, methodical pace. Enthusiastic cocksucking is always appreciated, but if you start slowly, you can save your energy for the finish, where it may be needed most. When your neck, arms, or jaw begin to ache, change positions. If the cramps in your neck or jaw become painful, pause to stroke him with your hand and give your mouth and neck a rest. You can also break up the action by taking a minute or two to lick his balls, kiss his thighs, perineum, or torso, or add a sex toy to your play. Be creative with your breaks. If you're in pain, or know that your neck is going to be complaining, plan ahead to use pillows for comfort or choose positions that don't require you to hold your head up, such as lying on your back with him straddling your chest.

Fellatio for Injured or Disabled People

An injury that impairs movement, comfort, or response to stimulation can affect the choices we make when fellatio is on the menu. When either you or your lover are physically limited in some way, sometimes a blow job is the best (or only) kind of sex play you can feasibly engage in—and we all know that most injuries, even painful ones, don't interfere with lust or horniness. Wanting to get off when you've got something you need to work around, such as a cast, a strained back, or limited privacy, just means you need to get a little more creative.

When you're hurting or limited in your movement, props, bolsters, and pillows are your erotic handmaidens. People with neck injuries should choose positions that support the head: sideways 69 with a pillow under your head, man on top, having him stand while you're seated, or sitting reverse in a high-backed chair with him on a higher surface. Folks with back injuries already know how pillows provide relief under their knees, and pillows can also go between the knees of whoever's hurting and lying sideways—let comfort in nonsexual situations be your guide. You may even end up on your back with your head and back piled on pillows, like a pasha, as your lover thrusts into your mouth, but if it feels good, who minds? Also, for back pain, make use of furniture such as low stools, which can be used bed-side—or anywhere, for that matter.

Men with disabilities will have varying capacities for receiving oral stimulation, but this depends on the type of disability and, if it is progressive, how far it has progressed. Needless to say, you should never consider a disabled man asexual—we're all pleasure-seekers, no matter what type of house we live in. Disabilities fit into various cate-gories: mobility, communication, deafness, vision impairment, or other diagnosed conditions such as multi-ple sclerosis, diabetes, or attention deficit disorder (ADD).

A man with multiple sclerosis might find genital stimulation pleasurable but may have difficulty achiev-ing orgasm, he may be combating fatigue, and erections may not be possible, or reliable—but do not assume that if he doesn't have an erection, he's not enjoying himself. The common mistake the medical community makes time and again when encountering *sex, men,* and *MS* in the same sentence is reducing everything to terms of erectile dysfunction. Let's toss yet another oversim-plification of male sexuality right out. MS is a disease of the central nervous system (brain and spinal cord), and it interferes with erections. It can cause numbing or tin-gling sensations in the genitals, difficulty feeling or achieving orgasms, and fatigue, and it can make focus-ing on stimulation difficult. Because it affects the pathways from brain to genitals, willed sexual response becomes less reliable; reflexive responses (involuntary erection, orgasm, sensation) can remain intact. And these things can change over time. Because some men with MS may experience pain during stimulation, communication about sex is essential. Some things may feel wonderful for a few weeks, then unpleasant for a while. Talking about how things feel to him, and becoming comfortable with talking about oral sex while you're doing it, makes oral sex better—and hotter.

Diabetes can also affect sexual functions; it's not unheard of for a man to see his doctor about erection issues only to discover he has diabetes. The reasons the disease interferes with his sexuality vary, but vascular disease (a frequent diabetes complication) can reduce blood flow and affect erection, neuropathy can cause nerve damage and reduce sensation, orgasm may become increasingly difficult to achieve, and ejaculation may not occur. Oral sex may still feel delightful; be sure to check in with him about varying your levels of stimulation.

ADD sufferers will find that their mind is racing uncontrollably when they want to be relaxing and enjoying fellatio—their brain is traveling at warp speed when they just want to sustain a fantasy, watch you work, or focus on orgasm. Treatment for ADD can help, but because many of the prescribed pharmaceuticals inhibit erection and/or orgasm, you should stress the importance of sexual functioning to your doctor before the prescription is written.

For some paraplegic and quadriplegic men, sexual function is impaired, but for others it's not impaired at all. Perhaps the fun is in finding out! If there is some impairment, it's possible that function and feeling can be increased over time—practice, anyone? After a spinal cord injury, the spinal center for sexual functioning is generally intact; it's the communication center from brain to spinal center that's usually disrupted. Unless some sensation in the area of his genitals remains, the usual sensation of orgasm is lost, and erections and ejaculation will be involuntary if they occur, though he may experience phantom orgasm elsewhere in his body. A playful, communicative partner makes all the difference in the world.

Keep Your Lipstick Perfect

Those of us who do our best to get through a cocktail party or dinner out while keeping lipstick a) on, and b) where it's supposed to stay—on our lips—have unique concerns when it comes to giving head. Of course, women in the movies go down, come up, and it's as if nothing happened. But when we try it in real life, it winds up looking like a car wreck between us and his cock. Fortunately for us, a higher power invented the drag queen.

Drag queens brought the technology of stay-put lipsticks from the theater to the streets. The best, though difficult to find, is a liquid used in the theater called Lip Set by Signature Solutions. You apply your lipstick (sorry, no gloss under or over), paint it on with the supplied brush, and let it dry. Then you have perfect lipstick that you can do anything with for four to six hours. There is a version of this same product from a different company, sold in drugstores, that comes in a roll-on applicator. It works for only about two hours, and sadly, your lipstick comes off right away when you give a blow job—due largely, I think, to the imprecise application of the roll-on. Some more commercially available options come from major cosmetic companies, sold under the heading of "stay put" lipsticks. These come in a variety of colors, and some can survive pretty heavy make-out sessions—perfect for our purposes. Cover Girl's Outlast was the best competitor for Lip Set, and I might add that the testing was rigorous.

How to Go Down on a Strap-On

Strap-on sex isn't just for breakfast anymore: not only are all types of people experimenting with strap-on sex, but they're not just using it for vaginal or anal penetration. *Strap-on sex* refers to having sex with a dildo and harness. You and your partner get a harness made to fit a dildo, and a dildo that's the size and shape of your preference, and one of you wears it during sex. The common conception is that only lesbian couples use strap-ons (and they do) but gay men also strap it on every now and then, and in increasing numbers, hordes of straight couples are adding strap-ons to their sex lives.

There are many contexts for strap-on use. In lesbian sex, strap-ons can be used to enhance fantasy play, to delineate roles, or simply for hands-free penetration. Gay men strap it on for the same reasons, but the harness is worn differently; either it is worn above the penis, or the harness has room for penis and testicles to hang freely. Straight men can employ a dildo and harness for a variety of reasons (for instance, erectile dysfunctions), or the female partner can wear the harness and penetrate her male lover in any context that turns the two of them on. Strap-ons are great whenever you want an extra erection, and they are highly erotic visually for both the wearer and the intended recipient.

Women or men who are inclined to give or receive head with a strap-on dildo may find that the subject brings up some interesting questions about their own (or their partner's) gender roles. Some folks find this titillating; swapping or sharing roles for a hot round of sex play opens whole new doors of sexual arousal and fantasy, which for some people is an aphrodisiac. However, others find that the very idea of opening these doors makes them uncomfortable. The notion of having the gender they identify with reshaped for a sexual fantasy may be felt as a challenge to who they are—at the very core of their being. For them, it's not okay to play with this stuff, and not fun to even think about it. If you find yourself accidentally stumbling across an emotional land mine, backtrack, be a supportive listener, and let it go. There are plenty of other ways to have fun with your lover.

Fellatio lends itself perfectly to strap-on sex. One look at your lover in a sexy harness, all buckles and straps, with an erect member jutting suggestively from their body, and it's difficult to resist the temptation to swallow them whole. Many of the same principles, tricks, and skills apply to fellating a dildo on your lover as to going down on an actual cock. You can create any context for the encounter you like: you can be in control and taking charge of that cock, or out of control and being used like a toy, you can demonstrate your naughty skills to your lover, or you can tenderly be making love to every inch of them. Reading up on techniques in other chapters of the book, such as types of strokes, controlling your gag reflex, or positioning, will give you a lot of the information you need when you go down. But the important difference in giving head to a strap-on is that you will approach the techniques you apply from a different angle: instead of being focused on the way the penis *feels*, you're focused on how the owner *sees* you.

When you suck strap-on cock, you're putting on a show, and making the wearer feel hot in that harness— and it's probably a big turn-on for you, too. See how you treat the dildo visually, and maintain plenty of eye contact, employ very visual oral techniques, and use your hands a lot. Your hands can roam, jerk the dildo off in your face, or grab your lover's hips to pull them into you, or they can stimulate the wearer beneath the harness (though you should make sure this is okay before you try it—some people don't want that type of stimulation, so ask permission first). The way you give head to a dildo is different for the reasons I just mentioned, but strap-on fellatio is also unique in that you aren't necessarily giving a blow job that ends with an orgasm. You're down there until you or your lover decide you're finished, or you both decide to switch activities.

Harnesses and dildos can be bought in adult sex toy stores, though for good quality and ease of use, you can find better toys in the more upscale shops, boutiques, and stores that cater to women (see chapter 13, "Resources," for stores). When choosing a harness, determine your price range, which material you'd like it made of (leather, fabric, neoprene), and how you'd like to wear it. Do you want an opening for access to your genitals, do you prefer a snug or very adjustable fit, do you want it to be easy to conceal beneath your clothes? Dildos come in more shapes, sizes, and colors than you can imagine, but be sure you purchase one made to be worn in a harness, and that it will fit into the harness you want. Dildos that can be worn with a harness have wide, circular bases to help them stay put. Most of the all-in-one strap-on units you'll find in mainstream adult toy stores are cheaply made and not worth your money—skip 'em. Read more about sex toys and materials in chapter 10, "More Techniques." One nice thing about purchasing the penis you're going to fellate is that you can practice in private before the main event—highly recommended!

Back Alley Baby

by Alison Tyler

"Do we want one made from neon pink jelly?" Chelsea murmurs. "Or a black-and-white marble swirl?"

I giggle as my lover points to a cock as long as my forearm. Wouldn't want to play hide-and-seek with that. Still, the crazier the space-age colors, the odder the textures, the wetter my panties. Who would have guessed that shopping for a sex toy would be this much of a turn-on? And it's not just because we're in a hip, sex-positive store surrounded by helpful salesgirls who look as if they wrote the manual on fucking. No, what really appeals to me is the same thing I find alluring about the Nordstrom shoe department: the outrageous selection. I mean, there are literally hundreds of different types of toys to choose from. We're not just talking length and girth, but colors, features, materials.

"How about that one?" Chelsea asks, obviously teasing as she indicates a monstrous devil-red number decorated with rounded bumps and a cynical smile.

I wonder who would choose a dildo like that, and suddenly, I'm no longer centered on the thought of the two us shopping for a sex toy. I'm lost in the thought of all the different people who have considered these items in the past, who have chosen the one they wanted and taken their precious treasures home to play with. What type of woman would like the dildo with the rabbit ears? Who would choose the double-headed U-shaped creation that can fill two holes at once?

"This one," Chelsea says finally, and I realize with a tightness in my chest that she's right. It doesn't actually look like a penis. Too smooth. Too perfectly rocket shaped. Too sapphire blue.

I nod and watch the sultry brunette sales chick pluck a box from a high-up shelf, handing over the toy and a harness to Chelsea in exchange for her credit card. Pussy, I think, be still. We have to get home before you can get served.

That admonition doesn't stop my clit from twitching or my cheeks from flushing neon-pink as Chelsea whispers in my ear. "You're going to get this nice and wet for me, aren't you, girl?"

"Mm hmmm."

"Wet with your hungry mouth."

"Mm hmmm," I say again.

"Wet back there in the alley—"

Now, I pause, but she doesn't. With a request spoken in undertone to the pierced sales dyke, she disappears behind a door that says Employees Only. When she returns, I immediately sense that something has changed. Her stride is different in her indigo boot-cut jeans. Her gray eyes are glowing. Empty-handed, she leads me in a pony-step out the door and around the corner. Presses me up against the chipped brick wall between two gray metal dumpsters, opens her fly with a single tug, and then pushes me down on my knees.

Dirty, my mind screams. Not X-rated dirty. Not sinful dirty. But filthy dirty. Crumpled newspapers wafting around us. Garbage smells. Creatures rustling unseen but heard.

"Suck it."

Working that luscious rod around in my mouth, I am transported. The toy is so blue, and smooth, and delicious as it slides between my lips that I forget everything else. In public, we are alone. My hot tongue slips up and down, tickling the tip, learning the curves. Deep throating something this silky smooth seems the most natural thing in the world. I go down, down, down on it. Fucking that toy with my mouth. Showing Chelsea exactly how much I want to please her.

"Get it really wet," my lover says, and now my mind is overwhelmed by a completely new—and very selfish—thought. How sweet this plaything will feel when it meets my cunt. "Get it wetter than wet," she whispers. "Wetter than me."

At her words I realize how aroused Chelsea is already. Putting one hand up to her gently rounded inner thighs, I stroke softly there as I suck on her. Christ, it's good. My fingers finding her swollen clit up under the harness and tapping on it as I keep up the steady ride with my mouth. My lips play tricks over the tip. My throat contracts. There is motion out at the end of the alley. Peripherally, I make out the blur of sunflower-yellow taxi cabs, the medley of colors as pedestrians crowd along the cracked concrete. But in my little world, there is only one thing: the blue, smooth sex toy between my parted lips.

"Get it all wet," Chelsea says. "Get it ocean wet."

I am. I know where it's going, and I know what to do. I want to feel this alien object probing my inner walls. But first, I want to suck and suck and suck. Why? I don't know. The hot pulse of sex in that store started me off. Chelsea's teasing glances as she played with all the different paraphernalia. And the fact that she chose the right toy without hesitation. Understanding that I didn't want real, I wanted cool.

But it's warm now. Warm from my wet mouth, as my pussy is warm in my cargo pants. Chelsea will take care of me. I have faith. When she's good and ready, she'll whip me around so my palms are splayed on the brick wall of the store, and she'll lower my slacks and slide aside my lacy lipstick-red thong, and thrust this space-age toy into my pussy.

For now, I do what she wants. Licking, sucking. Slurping on her hard blue rod, as only a back alley baby should.

Deep Throat

Possibly the most famous film of porn's golden age was the 1972 film *Deep Throat*, in which the adult actress Linda Lovelace made her most famous starring appearance. In the film, she played a woman who discovers with the aid of a very randy doctor that her clitoris is located in the back of her throat. Not a terribly complicated (or even possible) idea, but the plot device enabled the filmmaker to showcase Linda's amazing real-life talent for fellating a penis of any size all the way down into her throat. When the filmmaker originally witnessed her doing it in person, in his office, he was inspired to create the film.

When *Deep Throat* hit the theaters, Lovelace's performance caused such a stir that millions of Americans watched explicit sex onscreen for the first time. Frank

Sinatra, Spiro Agnew, Warren Beatty, Truman Capote, Nora Ephron, and Bob Woodward (who used Deep Throat as the name for his key Watergate source) saw the film on its first run, and eventually more people saw *Deep Throat* in theaters than any other adult film. *Deep Throat* brought hard core into popular culture and played for eight consecutive years at a theater in Hollywood. And the technique, or at least a name for it, entered our collective consciousness, changing our sexual cultural landscape.

In terms of pleasure and what constitutes an effective blow job, there are countless differing opinions of this technique. Because of its reputation, and because it seems like virtually every porn starlet can sword-swallow with ease, it is an oft-requested skill, and most folks who give head want to know how to do it. Yet, for as many men out there who want their partners to swallow their penis whole, there are an equal number who say that receiving deep throat pales in comparison to, say, having their balls tugged, or getting a fierce and enthusiastic blow job. People who like to perform the technique enjoy it wholesale, relishing that they can take him all the way down, get turned on by the idea and act, and feel incredibly sexy for having the skill. There are lovers who might only do it because their lover wants them to—a turn-on in its own right. Some consider it merely a novelty; others might think it's "the bomb." However you come to it, learning to deep throat can increase your ease and comfort with fellatio in general, and it's a terrific skill to add to your fellatio bag of tricks.

One of my favorite things to do is when he's all the way in I "milk" him with my tongue and

throat. I hold my head totally still; I can do this
and masturbate at the same time, which I always
want to do. He makes the most amazing noises!

Deep throating, novelty or not, can feel delicious to the recipient. The tip of your finger is a great place to begin understanding why—next time you're in the proximity of a chocolate cake, dip one of your fingers in the frosting and suck it off, using the front part of your mouth (lips and tongue). The tip is the most sensitive part of your finger, in the same way his penis is most sensitive at the head and along the underside. This feels really good, but see how your finger feels when you push it all the way in, down to the base (if you can). Your finger is completely surrounded by the warmth and wetness of your mouth. This is the allure and pleasure of deep throating. When you take him all the way in, he is completely engulfed by the pleasurable sensations of your mouth. And for some men, the act itself can be a fantasy-fulfilling turn-on, or an emotionally satisfying act of acceptance.

Learning the logistics of deep throating is half the battle. Familiarizing yourself with anatomy of the mouth and throat will give you an idea of what exactly is going on when his penis goes past the back of your tongue. Underlying your oral anatomy are the nerve responses that trigger pleasurable messages to your brain and also the dreaded gag reflex. Angles and positioning are key for comfort and sustaining the activity—yours and his— for any length of time. Breathing and rhythm are also a big part of the process, both of which work in tandem. Combine these elements with your own preferred tricks and techniques, and you'll be deep throating in ease, comfort, and pleasure.

The Anatomy of the Mouth and Throat

If you've never had any trouble with your mouth, you probably haven't given it much thought. Blowing kisses, licking ice cream, crunching popcorn, swallowing saliva,

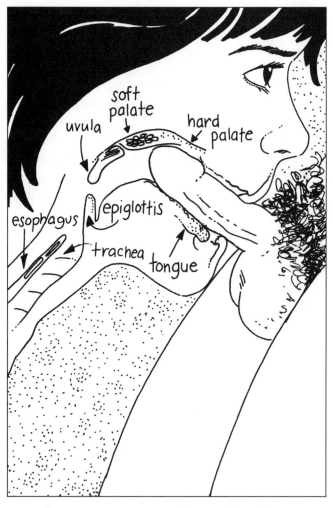

Illustration 10. Anatomy of the Mouth and Throat

talking a mile a minute—these things all happen with nary a conscious thought, like breathing. Our entire oral cavity is a system of constant motion, aqueous and in flux, a self-maintaining motion machine that performs numerous functions and is supported by hundreds of muscles, glands, and even helpful bacteria. Let our tour begin with a kiss.

Our lips are the first thing we meet: two soft and very sensitive membranes that line the opening of the mouth, the covering skin being somewhere between true skin and the moist mucous membrane that lines the inside of your mouth. The lips are made of muscle fibers interspersed with elastic tissues that are filled with hundreds of nerve endings, making them amazingly, deliciously sensitive. Beyond the lips are teeth, which should remain covered whenever possible throughout your oral sex session. The receptive and versatile tongue lines the bottom of your mouth, and it's another excellent tool in your oral sex arsenal and a means by which you can taste and erotically take in your lover's cock. On the front roof of the mouth is your hard palate, which flows into the back of your mouth to become the soft palate—these palates provide a firm backing for creating suction with your tongue and the seal of your lips. The soft palate is where the mouth ends and the throat begins.

It's crucial to understand where these two worlds of the mouth and throat meet, because deep throating is an act of swallowing. When you look into your throat, you can see the *uvula* hanging down; the area behind it is known as the *fauces*. The fauces rounds out the curvature in the back of your throat, arcing down and becoming the hidden pharynx, which continues unseen to your vocal cords. The pharynx is the transition between your throat and the openings of both windpipe (trachea) and esophagus. When you deep throat, your partner's penis (or strap-on) will travel this far.

Separating the windpipe and esophagus is an upright flap of cartilage called the *epiglottis*. This erect, yet flexible, matron guards both openings like a stern gatekeeper, taking cues from nerve responses about which direction to turn and either allow air in or out, or provide a passage for food and liquids to reach their proper destination, the stomach. Swallowing elicits the response of the epiglottis to lying against the windpipe, closing off air to the lungs for a momentary passing of fluids or fuel. To swallow anything, you have to stop breathing for a second, and to swallow a stiff cock you'll need to keep this in mind and time your breaths accordingly.

If something lingers in your pharynx for a moment too long, or if the object is large and/or hard, your body will intervene on your behalf and attempt to expel whatever is holding up the breathing by triggering your gag reflex. This is an involuntary nerve response, meaning that it happens without your thinking about it, and gagging is your body's defense against choking. The throat muscles constrict to push out the foreign object, and the constriction occasionally can (sometimes quickly, especially with repeated force from an object) trigger a vomit response. Gagging will make you salivate as well—saliva is like nature's own lube, so don't be embarrassed.

The gag reflex can be overcome, or at least worked around. Some people can control it quite easily. Some happy fellators even shrug and say, "What gag reflex?"—while many others contend with it occasionally obeying their wishes and other times not at all. There are a number of techniques you can employ during fellatio to move past the reflex and keep the action going, though it makes all the difference in the world if desire, arousal, and passion are driving your oral sex session. It's tough not to gag if you don't want to be going down on him. It's easier not to gag if you're really turned on.

Tips for Avoiding Gagging

I heard this from a gay guy: take a deep breath and hold it in. That stops the gag reflex.

You can sense the feeling of gagging as it comes on, and plan ahead with your response. Keeping your hand on his penis is essential; you can stave off deep thrusts that might trigger gagging by using your hand as a spacer. As your throat constricts, try the following suggestions:

- Back off and continue your strokes. Take a few deep breaths, and swallow. Then return to what you were doing.
- Try an alternating pattern with your mouth and hand: take him in your mouth and then back out for a few strokes of your hand, and repeat.
- If possible, move the head of his penis to the front of your mouth and hold still for a moment until the feeling passes.
- Remember to breathe while going down; this helps a lot.
- Give yourself regular breaks from having him in your mouth; this is especially helpful if you gag easily.
- Practice on a dildo or penis-sized vegetable before you go down, and learn to work with your gag reflex.

- Explore any psychological reasons you might be impelled to gag. If the sex act, sex in general, or his genitals are offensive to you, explore why you might be feeling this way. Learn as much as you can about what bothers you, and if you aren't ready for this, then reconsider performing oral sex until you are ready.
- Don't go down on him if you're already feeling ill, or have consumed drugs or alcohol that may make you feel queasy. Some prescription drugs can make you feel nauseated and will make your gag reflex extra sensitive.
- Shift the angle at which his penis is entering your mouth. Many people say that coming down on him from above is easier; try having him lie down or sit, with you facing his feet.
- If you need a break but don't want to take him out of your mouth, shift the angle of his penis from the back of your throat to your cheek.
- Use arousal to decrease the gag reflex. It does wonders!

The biggest obstacle is the gag reflex. Some of it is psychological, but some is physiological. If I tune in to my arousal primarily, it helps me overcome that reflex.

If I relax, take a slow deep breath, and take it bit by bit, it works. I have to get my throat used to it. It eventually slides right in.

It helps to make sure he doesn't thrust. I have to do all the moving.

When you deep throat a penis or dildo, you are swallowing it all the way past the opening of your throat. What's more, you're not just putting it in there for a second before it's over—you're giving head, so it's going to be pushing down your throat over and over. The only way to be able to do this is to overcome your gag reflex through practice. Famous magician Harry Houdini was a master of his own gag reflex. Magicians are physical performers who practice physical acts over and over until they seem effortless, and Houdini did exactly this with his throat. He would use the back of his throat as a hiding place for objects, putting them in his mouth and holding them easily in his throat, then bringing them back up when he needed them. Don't try this at home, kids—but what I am suggesting is that with practice, anything is possible, and this is very true of conquering the urge to gag.

Practice First

Practice on a dildo—anything similar in size and shape to the penis you intend to deep throat is good, or get something as close to realistic as you can (if you'll be giving head to a guy; if you will be fellating another dildo, then pick a similar one). Do not use anything that will break and possibly choke you, like a banana, and do not use anything that could slip from your grasp when it's in your throat—for deep throat practice, cucumbers and zucchinis are out.

Make sure you always have a hold on the dildo; dildos with a base you can grab onto are recommended, because you can use the base like a handle and not worry about it going too deep, and you can easily back it out if you panic. Insert it into your mouth, and gradually let yourself get comfortable with the way it feels. With a gentle in-and-out motion, slowly push it a little farther back each time. Ease it in as far as feels comfortable to you, and remember to breathe around the dildo. When it reaches a certain point it will be difficult to take a breath, and it's easy to panic—as it goes deep into your throat, you'll want to exhale before you push it in, then inhale when you pull it out. Use this breathing technique when you deep throat your lover. Experiment with the sensation of swallowing with the dildo in your throat, and try a few practice thrusts as you become more comfortable. Practice every day until you feel confident to try it in real life.

> *I start by placing it near the back of my throat, and then by degrees, I swallow more. I find after awhile that I am able to bypass the gag reflex. It's best not to deep throat him on a full stomach, also.*

> *I've always found it works best with him lying down or leaning back, and to kneel beside him approaching him perpendicularly. I find that if I am sitting, I can't get the angle right and have to be on my knees (unless he is really narrow, which makes it all-around easier). Sometimes it works better if I am facing the opposite direction pointing toward his feet—it's all about positioning for me.*

> *The best deep throat blow job I have ever received was when this girl hung her head over the side of the bed. I am over 7 inches and she took it all down her throat all the way to my balls. I couldn't believe it.*

Certain positions are conducive to opening up your throat, which makes deep throating easier. When you're on your knees facing him, his penis is going to wind up pointing upward toward the soft palate in the back of your throat—right where it will trigger the strongest gag reflex. Angling his cock down your throat (not toward the top of your mouth) is the most comfortable way to deep throat and will make you gag the least. The best position is lying on your back, with your head tilted back and slightly off the edge of a bed or couch. Try it, and you'll see how it elongates your neck and throat. Approaching the penis from above is also easier on your palate, and many people report that the angle of insertion is excellent for deep penetration. Another good position is 69 (reciprocal oral sex); you are essentially approaching from above, and the pathway down your throat is straightened.

Breathing, or remembering to breathe, is another essential component of deep throating (and not gagging). Time your up and down strokes with your breath. Inhale as you draw him in; exhale as you pull him out. It will almost seem as if you were breathing him in, a sexy notion itself. The best place to see breathing techniques in action is in porn; *Deep Throat* is a great example.

An Aphrodisiac for the Orally Fixated

People who deep throat may already have a handle on the link between their arousal and taking him all the way down—many find that deep throating turns them on like nothing else. There are two primary arousal sources stemming from deep throating: the physical stimulation, including the arousal hormones that are released, and the mental stimulation, encompassing the realms of fantasy fulfillment and desire. Some people find it turns them on so much, and so reliably, that it's their favorite sex act, period.

Your mouth is an erogenous zone, no question about it—but in its entirety. The back of your mouth, tongue, palate, and throat have a different range and number of nerve endings than the sensitive front of your mouth, but they transmit messages of pleasure to your brain (and genitals) just the same. Sucking (suckling) and swallowing in an erotic context stimulates nerve pathways whose function is to build on your arousal levels, including increasing the production of the arousal hormone, oxytocin. We get physical gratification from oral stimulation, and we get it in spades when we swallow our lover to the root. The intimacy of the complete face-to-penis contact inherent in deep throating is overwhelmingly hot. This encompasses all the other stimulating sensory information, such as seeing him up close and smelling his skin and pubic hair. The physical eroticism of deep throating can't be found anywhere else in the realm of sex. The physical sensory information is overwhelming, and it combines easily with the mental stimulation stemming from the act—physical and mental stimulation being required to work in tandem to produce arousal and orgasm. The reality of deep throating is right there in your face, and this is an incredible turn-on for many of us. Merely the fact (and realization) that you're doing it is hot—you're directly anchored to the moment, fully present. In addition, your fantasy life can be anywhere when you've got him in your throat. You can imagine that you're in a roomful of people, in public, a porn star, or anything else that turns you on.

Taking Deep Throat Further

Now that you've got the technique in your bag of tricks, know all there is to know about how and why it works, and know how to use it to turn yourself on, take your technique as far as it can go. There are a number of tricks and twists on the technique that can help you to heighten the experience for both of you. You'll likely come up with several of your own along the way, but here are some suggestions:

- When he's in deep, freeze, and swallow.
- Instead of moving your head, constrict your throat muscles around his penis, making the rhythmic movement occur within you.
- Put him all the way in and vary your rhythm with long and short strokes: alternate short and deep for a few beats, then long and deep for a few.
- Swallowing the head of his cock, twist your head slightly and slowly from side to side.
- Experiment with extending your tongue out the front of your mouth. It will rub the sensitive underside of his shaft.
- When you exhale, moan to vibrate him in your mouth.
- To give your hands something to do, cup, fondle, or tug on his balls, stimulate his perineum with your fingertips, penetrate his anus with your fingers or a sex toy. You can also reach up and play with his nipples.
- Grab his hips and bring him into your mouth, "forcing" him all the way in.
- Put his hands on your head. He can rest them lightly and enjoy feeling your head move in addition to the

fellatio, or he can move your head as he likes. It might turn you both on to have him "use" your head and mouth in this way. An adventurous variation is for him to grab fistfuls of your hair.

Oral Authority

by Alison Tyler

"I'm going to teach you how to suck cock," Audrey assured me after I confessed my lack of expertise in that particular sexual arena. I looked over at my beautiful blonde best friend, then let my gaze wander down to the crotch of her chicly faded 501s. She caught the glance and knew exactly what I was thinking. "Not on me, silly," she explained, "on Duncan." When I remained silent, she glanced up at me from her velvet sofa, her startling green eyes opened wide. "You do like Duncan, don't you, Stella?"

Now, I blushed. Duncan was Audrey's very attractive roommate. He had a regular spot on one of those beach-babe shows, and his body was just incredible. Tanned. Muscular. Perfect for the lifeguard he played on TV. Aside from that, he was actually an extremely nice guy. The thought of using him as a living sex toy both excited and terrified me.

"Why not start me off with a banana?" I asked, twirling one of my caramel-colored curls around my fingertips.

"Bananas break," Audrey said knowingly. "You don't want to choke. If anything, we can use a cucumber to get you ready while we wait for Duncan to show up."

Before I could say a word, she headed to the kitchen. I heard her rustling around in the refrigerator, and we she came back, she had a slender zucchini in one hand. "We were all out of cukes. So hold this while I buzz Duncan." That said, she dashed off a quick message to her roommate on his Blackberry, and then she returned to cuddle next to me on her leopard-print lounge. I sat staring at the vegetable and wondering why I was getting so wet.

"Here's the deal," Audrey began. "Breathing is the most important part of going down deep. Before you slide the zucchini into your throat, I want you to exhale—"

Her instructions reminded me of my Yoga class. Don't breathe the breath, let the breath breathe you. Still, I did my best, pretending the veggie was Duncan and slipping the head into my mouth. As I worked the slippery zucchini farther in, Audrey continued, "Inhale when you pull it out, and you'll be ready for him to slide inside you again." I pushed the smooth veggie-tool back into my throat, and I tentatively tried swallowing down on it. Quickly, I pulled the zucchini back out again.

"It feels weird," I said, hoping I didn't sound too panicked.

"You need the real thing," Audrey assured me. "But don't worry, I'll never leave your side. What you require in this sort of situation is an oral authority." I stared down at the slippery zucchini discarded despondently in my lap. "Giving head is just like anything else," Audrey continued. "You learn the little tricks of the trade, and your confidence grows. Duncan will be gentle with you. Just keep your hand on the base of his cock, and you'll be in control. You can push back if he's going too fast."

Duncan arrived ten minutes later. I wondered how many red lights he'd run on his way over, but I didn't bother asking. My face was probably as crimson as my dress, and I found that I couldn't meet his eyes. He sat down on the chair across from me and just smiled, obviously waiting for someone to tell him the game plan. Audrey perched her lithe body up on the arm of his chair and started whispering to him. I could make out snippets of her discussion—"Not a virgin, just not super comfortable with the whole idea"—and then I looked down at my hands again.

After a moment, Duncan came to sit by my side. "Is it something you really want to learn, Stella?" he asked.

I nodded.

"Then it's best to practice with friends," and the Cheshire grin on his face let me know he understood just how ridiculous this all was. A willing girl was going to give him a blow job, and he would be expected to give instructions all the way through. "But I'd like it if Audrey would help you relax, first," he said, and as he spoke, my naughty best friend got into position on the floor between my thighs and lifted the hem of my dress. As soon as I felt Audrey's breath on my panties, I sighed. And as soon as I sighed, Duncan put my hand on the crotch of his jeans. We were starting from the top.

Slowly, I worked down his button fly. Then I watched as he split the jeans open for me, revealing his erection. Audrey had her mouth pressed against my pussy now through my panties, and I turned my head and opened my own mouth, bringing the tip of Duncan's hard-on between my lips. "That's the way," he said, sliding his hands through my light brown curls. "You just relax and take it all the way down. The key word here is relax, and remember to breathe—"

I swallowed against the smooth, silky skin of his cock, then drew the length farther down my throat. As I worked him harder, Audrey continued her kissing and licking games between my legs. Suddenly, I realized that she wasn't simply working to build my arousal, she was showing me how I was supposed to tease Duncan. Closing my eyes, I paid attention to Audrey's lesson. I swirled my tongue around the shaft of Duncan's cock, then closed my lips firmly on the head. When Audrey tricked the tip of her tongue in a circle around my clit, I did the same thing to the head of Duncan's cock. And when she brought her hands into the action, cradling my hips and lifting up, I slid one hand down to cup and stroke Duncan's balls.

"Oh, yeah," he moaned, "just lightly. Just like that."

But what I really wanted to do was learn how to swallow. This had always made me back off from going down on a man. The not knowing what would happen frightened me too much to ever remain calm. My throat would close down, and I'd pull away and shake my head. Now, as Audrey continued to dine on me, I felt a wave of excitement transplant my previous fear. Duncan brought one hand against my throat, and he stroked there. "Relax," he said. "Relax and just let it happen. If you need to pull back for a second, that's okay."

At his instructions, I felt myself open up, felt his cock slip a little farther down my throat. Duncan sped up the rhythm now, sliding back and forth, gaining a bit of headroom with each thrust. It was as if he were fucking all the way through me, and that thought turned me on even more. As I grew more aroused, I worked him with a fiercer intensity. My fingers tripped down behind his balls, and I caressed that magical spot back there, danced the tips of my fingers more firmly against his skin. Duncan continued to help me now, thrusting deeper and deeper into my throat. I had to move to get more comfortable, and I pulled away from Audrey and went on all fours on the sofa, facing Duncan, drinking him.

Immediately, Audrey got behind me on the sofa, and she slid my panties down my thighs and squirmed her way back into a position that allowed her to go to work on my pussy once again. And as she brought me right to the peak, Duncan started to come. I could tell when it was going to happen by the way his moans grew louder, his breathing harsher. He gripped his hands onto my shoulders, held tight, and shot his load deep down my throat. I swallowed against him, draining every last drop, and then slowly he slid from my lips and collapsed back against the sofa.

Pulling away from Audrey, I sprawled next to him. I could taste his juices still, the tart taste of come, slightly salty, very sexy. When I flicked my tongue over my top lip, Duncan gave me one of his trademark smiles. "See?" he murmured, reaching out to stroke my hair out of my eyes. "Now, you're an oral authority as well."

I looked at him, then looked over at my green-eyed friend, whose mouth was shiny with my own erotic juices. "Time to share the pleasure," I told Duncan as we both reached for Audrey and spread her out on the couch...

10

More Techniques

Fellatio has this lovely, Zen-like way of being able to flow in and out of a wide variety of sexual activities. You can make it the only thing you do with your lover, a hands-and-mouth-only encounter, you can pepper it into your regular intercourse routine—or you can really spice things up by combining it with sex toys, penetration, or more. Pressure points can be stimulated to bring him to higher points of ecstasy, using the sensations of heat and cold can enhance pleasure, and you can try mixing pain with pleasure, adding bondage, or fantasy play to push the boundaries of fellatio.

Sex Toys

As we come to realize that we adults really like to be big kids sometimes, and that oral sex is one of the areas in which we can really be playful, then it's only natural for the fellatio discussion to turn to sex toys. The world of sex toys is big (and sometimes overwhelming), and there are quite a few you can add to fellatio, or use to enhance certain aspects of your stimulation.

Cock Rings

A cock ring is a ring worn around the penis and testicles to apply a steady pressure around the base, slightly restricting the blood flow to the penis. Not for all (but enjoyed by many), cock rings provide a continuous squeeze to his penis and testicles that can make any stimulation feel more pleasurable. The universally recognized cock ring style is a single leather band with snaps. It goes over the top of the penis's base and continues around and behind the testicles. Cock rings do not help with erectile difficulties, but many men say they help their erections last longer—however, this is different for everyone. But cock rings do have a nice way of pushing everything out and up...making a nice visual when you're up close and personal.

There are different types and styles of cock rings. They come in leather, fabric, neoprene, and various plastics and rubbers, and not all have snaps. Some snap, others fasten with Velcro, tie, or have sliding closures, and some are just rubber rings that stretch wide and slip on. A whole selection of complicated and torturous cock rings is available, and if your guy likes extra pressure or feelings of intense constriction when he's sliding in and out of your mouth, you can find cock rings with multiple straps, ball stretchers, ball dividers, or D-ring attachments for weights, ties, or leashes. Start with a single, simple ring, and see if he likes it.

Unless you're experienced with cock rings, never use rings that are metal or aren't stretchy enough to remove easily. These rings can come off only when he ejaculates or his erection subsides, which means icing him down if he panics or experiences pain or discomfort. Needless to say, if he experiences pain or discomfort when using a cock ring, remove the ring immediately.

Cock rings are easiest to apply and remove on men who trim or shave their pubic hair, but that's not required. Just keep an eye on hair that can get snagged when removing a stretchy rubber ring.

Vibrators

Do men really like vibrators? You bet. Some men like them a lot, and for these guys you can pick up a vibe and add it to your oral feast. Choosing what to use depends on what you have in mind. There are vibrators on the market for just about every scenario you can imagine, though you can always use any type of vibe in a pinch.

Men who like vibration have preferences as to how intense, where, and when in their pleasure cycle they like it. When you're not sure, ask him or have him show you. Generally speaking, vibration right on the head of his penis might feel too intense—popular spots where men like vibration are underneath the head, along the underside of the shaft (possibly at the base), and on their testicles, perineum, or anus. Access is easiest when he is lying on his back. You can easily hold his penis in your mouth and vibrate the underside of the shaft, run the vibe over his balls, or push farther south if he's game. For more on anal penetration, see the section later in this chapter.

Vibrators come in a kaleidoscopic assortment. You can buy them in penis shapes, whale shapes, smooth curves, or bumpy rides. You can find small ones that can be worn on the tip of your finger—perfect for fellatio, but don't insert them anywhere. Some are flared at the base for anal penetration and can be worn in strap-on harnesses. Vibrators also come with variations on speed and motion; some are made for penetration, while others are not. Vibrators are generally made of hard plastic or rubber blends: jelly rubber, clear or opaque, and quite porous; Cyberskin, lifelike, and extremely porous; vinyl, in flat colors, and not porous; and silicone, in many opaque colors, completely nonporous, and sterilizable. Porous models hold bacteria (which they pick up a lot of when used for penetration), so it's best to use these with condoms or toss them after a few uses—which is why they're inexpensive, and silicone fetches high prices. Hard plastic is nonporous.

Some vibrators vibrate, some pulse; they can have many speeds, dials, or just one or two speeds. When in doubt, buy a vibe with variable speeds, since a one-speed model may not necessarily be at the right speed for you or your partner; you can adjust the vibration intensity on these as you go. There are also insertable and noninsertable vibrators: all insertables are on a shaft of some kind, with no openings that would allow moisture to enter. No, you won't get shocked, but moisture would ruin your toy. Noninsertable vibrators, such as "egg" vibrators and Silver Bullets, are smaller and have cords attached. Never insert these and think you can tug on the cord to get them out—all battery-operated vibes are cheaply made, and you will just yank the cord out, leaving the vibe in. Electric vibrators are more reliable but also more expensive, and they almost always have only two speeds. Vibrators that can be worn on fingers are fantastic for fellatio—you just let your fingers do the walking while you lick—but don't insert these, either. Waterproof vibes are a good option, because they can take all the juices you can throw at them and they clean up easily in the sink, with no worry about getting water in the wrong areas.

Dildos and Harnesses

Dildos are sex toys used for penetration that do not vibrate. They're usually phallic-shaped, though you can find them in rocket shapes, whale shapes, and goddess images, or fashioned to represent objects d'art. They come in all shapes and sizes, a mind-boggling palate of colors, and a huge variety of materials. Made of everything from silicone to Cyberskin and Lucite to polished wood, dildos run the gamut of style and form. Most dildos that you find in women-run and boutique sex toy shops have a base, meaning a flat, circular end that allows you to stand them up, erect and proud. The base isn't just for display; it's usually there to make the dildo harness-compatible for those who want to engage in strap-on sex. Not all dildos have bases; some have a set of wrinkly balls to add a (perhaps ironic) touch of realism. A dildo can be used manually during fellatio—using it to penetrate him while you give him head—he can use it on himself, or one of you can wear the dildo in a harness while the other fellates. Read more about going down on a strap-on in chapter 8, "Any Way You Want It."

Harnesses can be worn by lovers of any gender for fun with strap-on fellatio. When selecting a harness, consider the look, fit, and functionality of the harness you'd like to wear. Most harnesses come in black, but you can find them in specialty shops in pink, blue, red, and white leather, glittery neoprene, or colored rubber. You'll find them in soft, buttery leathers, cool rubber, wetsuit material (neoprene), fabric, and Spandex. Skip the prepackaged dildo and harness kits and spend the extra dollars on separate items from women-run shops; the prepackaged sets are cheaply made, and their quality is unpredictable. Next, consider how you want to wear your dildo. Ask yourself if you want access to your genitals. Harnesses come in two main styles: two-strap (with the straps lying in the crease between your genitals and thighs) or single-strap (like a G-string panty). However, you can also find harnesses that fit in other styles, like bicycle shorts. Last, make sure that your harness will fit your dildo. The center ring may not be the same size as the dildo you select, and this could make a carefully planned evening a disappointment.

Anal Penetration

> Most guys I've been with go nuts when I grab their butt cheeks in both hands when they're in my mouth. This way you can also see how he might like having his butt hole touched.

> Touching his asshole when I go down on him is like pressing a magic button to make him come.

For me, finding out that my male lover likes anal penetration is like eating ice cream when you haven't had it in a really long time. Penetration is one of those very amazing things that connects you with your lover like nothing else, and it can be an incredible turn-on for both of you. With your finger or fingers, a dildo, or a vibrator, you enter into a realm of pleasure that is as deep for him as it is intimate for both of you. And in some men it's like hitting a pleasure switch—even the lightest touch on the outside of the anus sweeps some men straight to orgasm.

Many men (though not all) enjoy penetration during fellatio—that is, as long as you don't stop or interrupt the blow job. Fingers are wonderful to penetrate with, and as opposed to sex toys, they afford you the most feeling and movement. You'll already have your hands on him caressing and adding to your oral encounter, and when he's turned on you can experiment with massaging his buttocks and caressing the crack between his cheeks. If he responds positively, try slowly sliding a finger over the opening to his anus while you're giving him head. Be sure your hands are clean (read: scrubbed—no dirt or grime under your nails) and your fingernails are trimmed and filed smooth. Make sure you don't have any tiny cuts or hangnails.

If you've talked to him about penetration beforehand, you've got it under control and are way ahead of the game. Discussing anal play before you try it is advised, unless you and your lover already have sexual adventure and exploration on the table. Anal play for someone who's not ready for it can be very unsettling; don't guess how he might react, because for some guys, anal penetration is going too far. So, how do you add anal penetration to oral sex and make it pleasurable? Follow the three golden rules: go very slowly, listen to the person you're penetrating, and use lots of lube.

If you know he's into penetration, and he is at the point when he's not sure if he should be thrusting into your mouth or bucking onto your hand, check your accessories. You should have plenty of lube, and gloves or finger cots. The anus is an unlubricated area; it does not self-lubricate like a mouth or vagina, and the skin is thin enough to abrade easily. Use lube, lots of lube. You can never have too much lubricant. Use a thick, water-based lube. For smooth hands and to avoid getting bacteria from the anus on your hands, have a latex (or nonlatex nitrile or polyurethane) glove at the ready, or already on. Gloves also provide a firm, slippery sensation that feels absolutely delicious on the delicate anal tissues.

With the flat of your finger, or fingers, press lightly on the opening and hold it there. Increase the pressure a little, massaging and pressing in circular motions. Go very slowly, and listen to his cues or verbal instructions—for some, simply having their anus touched is all it takes to push them over the edge. Pay attention to lubrication, and never rely on saliva. In porn films they make it look like that's all they use, but that's not the case—they just don't show you the anal suppositories and numerous applications of lube.

Move your flattened fingers in a circular motion, and begin experimenting with penetration by pressing one well-lubed finger at the base of the opening (toward his tailbone). Massage the opening's base, and ask him if he wants you to go farther. Slowly slide your finger in up to the first joint (about an inch), and hold it there for a few breaths. You'll feel the ring of muscles around his opening squeeze and contract—just stay still as the muscles relax.

When you feel the muscles relax, slide your finger in slowly a little bit more, then back out, doing a gentle in-and-out, not all the way in yet. Once again, this may be all it takes for him to come, or to decide that it's not what he wants right now—but if he does want more, following his directions and body language from here, you can progress to more stimulation. You can go deeper or faster, or even add more fingers—but the rule of thumb is to do everything so slowly that you can practically feel the seasons changing around you. Anal penetration hurts when you go too fast, you don't use enough lube, the recipient isn't relaxed, or he doesn't really want to be doing it.

Once he's anally warmed up and ready for more penetration, you can bring anal sex toys into the picture. Sex toys used for anal penetration must have a flared base, meaning a base that prevents them from being pulled into the anal canal, where they can get lost—a nightmare waiting to happen. The sphincter muscles have minds of their own and like to squeeze and contract at will; we cannot control them. This serves to push and pull things in and out of the anus, and once something gets pulled in, there's no guarantee you're going to get it out without a trip to the hospital—which is what you'd have to do to prevent serous injury if, say, a hot, battery-powered vibrator went AWOL. Take a look at a standard butt plug and you'll see exactly what a flared base should look like. Buy toys that are safe for anal use, and don't get cute with carrots.

Vibrators can feel fantastic on the ass during fellatio, and you can tease and penetrate while you suck. The thing to know about vibrators and anal stimulation is that the outer third of the anus, and the prostate, contain more nerve endings than the anal canal and respond best to touch and vibration. The inner portion, inside the canal, has fewer nerve endings near the skin's surface and responds to feelings of fullness, pressure, and rhythm.

So, a vibrator will feel intense (intensely good) around the opening and the prostate area. But the vibration won't be a factor deep inside—the size, shape, and motion of the vibe will. To maximize your buzz, select insertable vibrators that have the vibration located at the base. When bringing a vibe into the action, start on the lowest speed, and give him more as he asks for it.

Squirt liberal amounts of lube on any toy you use, and reapply frequently. You can fuck the daylights out of him anally with a dildo he likes. Or, insert a butt plug and keep it in place while you suck and bring him to orgasm; just don't leave it in for extended periods, or it will get downright uncomfortable. Chances are good that his PC muscles will squeeze the plug out before he orgasms; if you like, you can hold it in place with your free hand. It can also get forced out during orgasm, which is an okay way to remove it. But if it's big and stays in place, after he comes ask him to take a few deep breaths and let him know you are going to remove the plug on an exhale—then remove it on the second or third exhale.

The Prostate

In men, anal stimulation and penetration can crank up the arousal for a variety of reasons, some psychological and some physical. One big, or little, reason is that rising star on the stage of sex play, the prostate gland. Much ado has been made about the prostate, and this tiny celebrity of the glandular glitterati doesn't show any signs of slowing down as men and their partners discover the erotic potential of prostate stimulation.

In most every sex book you'll pick up, if you can find a reference to the prostate gland at all (without it being exclusively related to cancer), you'll notice a few strange things about the way authors tend to deal with the subject. Some impart a homophobic tone that makes even me wonder if I'm repressing anything—and this goes for both male and female authors. It's as if they wanted you to be absolutely sure they're straight when they're telling you about what's inside guy's butts, and that you are too, and that everyone's still straight after they read about it. The concept of male anal penetration obviously carries a lot of stigma and shame for these authors. This would be funny, if it weren't so frustrating trying to get information out of their texts. The other unfortunate thing most books do when they cover real-life, try-this-at-home prostate stimulation (which is rare) is rush through the material and present it in a cold context, as if no one would really try this during sex. The gay guides are straightforward and enthusiastic, but there aren't many of them available. And the straight manuals never suggest that the man try to find the prostate for himself—especially during masturbation, which is something I highly recommend. Oh, and did I mention that prostate play, or the enjoyment thereof, has nothing to do with sexual orientation? It doesn't. End of discussion.

The prostate gland is located at just about the center of the male urogenital system, inside the perineal wall. It sits just below the bladder, producing the fluid that mixes with semen in ejaculate, and is connected to the urethra, the muscles that line the perineum, and the sphincter muscle. If there's an epicenter to male orgasm, then this must be it. For a thorough understanding of prostate anatomy and location, see chapter 2, "The Anatomy of a Man's Pleasure." Many men, though not all, find that when they're aroused, prostate stimulation is intensely pleasurable; that's because the nerve pathway form the brain to the penis runs through the rectum, and one large nerve bundle is located just beneath the prostate. Additionally, the root of the penis is more or less anchored at the prostate, so when you massage the prostate you also transmit sensation to the base of his penis.

The gland is rounded, shaped like a walnut, but slightly cleaved down the center so it has a furrowed seam and two subtle halves that can be felt with the pad of your finger (when touched from inside the anus). In size it can be anywhere from the size of a small chestnut to a large walnut, or even larger in men over forty. When he's aroused, it swells and becomes firm to the touch, and it's a lot easier to feel it. Plus, it's much more fun to touch when he's hot and bothered.

Begin your prostate explorations when he's good and ready; the prostate is easier to find when he's aroused, and he will enjoy the touch more at this point. You can stimulate his prostate externally, through the perineum, or internally, by inserting a finger, dildo, or butt plug into his anus. External stimulation is done by massaging or applying gentle pressure to his perineum, on the area near, but not on, the anal opening. See if he likes this; not all men do, and some might find it downright uncomfortable. Try vibration, and see how that feels, too.

Penetration is the most direct way to stimulate the prostate. The preceding section has all the information you need on the importance of lubrication, patience, communication, and safety—follow the rules! But prostate stimulation differs slightly, because you focus your attention on the gland rather than on the fullness, pressure, or rhythm you're applying to his rectum. When he's aroused and ready for penetration, take the necessary steps to pleasurably insert your finger, then slightly curve it toward the front of his body: facing him (perhaps with his penis in your mouth or other hand), make a come-hither stroking motion with your finger. Don't poke, push, or stab forward. The gland is delicate, and because of its positioning, some men report the sensation of having to pee when it's stimulated. That's a feeling that some men don't like at all, and you may wind up switching activities if he's uncomfortable. If he experiences any pain when his prostate is touched, he should have it checked by his doctor.

Apart from possibly making him feel like peeing, touching his prostate will certainly make him feel a full-ness and pressure that he can feel in his penis. Juicy men who are prone to leaking pre-come may leak a lit-tle more when you massage their prostate; that's because the prostate is where the fluid comes from. Massage it gently but firmly; you can simply move your finger in the come-hither motion, or you can keep your curved finger stiff and move it in and out. As he gets close to orgasm the gland will swell more, and it will get quite hard before he ejaculates. The orgasms from prostate stimulation are often described by men as deep, intense, and powerful.

Rimming

Rimming, or analingus, is kissing, caressing, or penetrat-ing your lover's anal opening with your tongue. For many people, rimming is a delicious experience, on both the giving and the receiving end. Some say there is nothing as arousing as having their lover's warm, soft tongue and lips give them pleasure in such an incredibly intimate place, and those who love to give it find the experience equally arousing. Also, the feeling of doing something taboo or "dirty" heightens the experience for some. Because the delicate pucker of the anus is packed with sensitive nerve endings, rimming can be all it takes to push someone over the orgasmic edge.

For men, rimming adds a new spectrum of pleasure to the sexual experience. A fantastic blow job can include delicate licks and flutters of the tongue on and around the anus, and rimming can be a great introduction to the sensation of anal penetration. For men who enjoy being penetrated, this is a delicious tease for the main course to come, and for men who aren't sure about penetration, rimming allows them to comfortably try out the sensation of anal stimulation to see if they might like it.

The easiest position for rimming is doggie-style, with the rim-ee on all fours. This lets you gently spread his cheeks with your hands, and see everything clearly as you dip your tongue in and out. If he has a lot of hair down there, this position is optimal for parting the furry seas—and if this notion makes you uncomfortable, let it be known that everyone has hair down there. If you do not naturally have hair around your anus, you are either a) too young to be reading this, b) shaving or waxing it, or c) a genetic anomaly. Doggie-style licking is ideal because it also provides a fantastic rear view of his testicles, which you can squeeze, rub, and pull on as you lick. Also, you can pull his erect penis back between his legs for reverse cocksucking, though some men find this uncomfortable. When in doubt, ask how it feels.

With the delicate pucker of the anus in full view, gently kiss and lick his cheeks as they slope inward toward the crack. Work your way closer into the furrow, taking your time to let him get used to the sensation—or to tease him if you know he likes it. You can make your first touch in various ways:

- Lick the entire furrow from top to bottom as you would an ice-cream cone, with a big, flat tongue.
- With softened lips, kiss it directly, over and over.
- Press your flattened tongue against the opening and hold it, then slowly start to move it in up and down, or give him an in-and-out massage.
- With the very tip of your tongue, lightly lick in a ring around the rim of the opening—"rimming" him.

You can start with one of these and then try them all out to see what he likes. When you find something that makes him moan, groan, and push his butt in your face, stay with it for a few minutes. Gradually, work your tongue into a rhythm with a short, firm lick. Continue the beat for a while: this should get him pretty aroused. If you decide you want to go a step further, begin darting your tongue in as you lick, graduating to what's called "tongue-fucking." Moan your appreciation and see how he responds—moaning vibrates your tongue and simulates a vibrator. When you want him to explode, slide a lubed hand onto his cock and jack him off while you lick—there's no sensation in the world like it.

A man with lower back pain or mobility issues can simulate the doggie position by lying on his stomach with pillows under his hips, comfortably raising his butt for optimal licking. Having him lie stomach-up with pillows under his butt is also an option, though you have to spread his legs quite wide for access. In this position, placing pillows under his knees can help ease strain on his back. Lying sideways may be comfortable, too; he'll want to put a pillow between his legs for the lower back, and the pillow will also serve to keep his legs slightly spread—though he may eventually end up on his stomach as you pull his cheeks apart.

Cleanliness is often the number one concern for would-be rimmers and rim-ees alike. Taking a nice long shower or bath beforehand is always recommended, and you can bathe together to make it part of the seduction. If your partner is reluctant because of cleanliness issues, begin rimming in the shower, where you'll both make everything squeaky-clean. Men who are comfortable with enemas can have one before showering and know they're clean from the inside out.

Flavored lubricants are an option for people who want to try rimming but shudder at the notion of tasting their lover's natural flavors, though they come with several caveats. Flavored lubes taste awful, even the lime, kiwi, or piña colada versions. Because they're packed with sugar, they are not an option for diabetics or other people who don't tolerate the effects of sugar well. But they do their job to some extent, transforming the eager anus into an artificial-raspberry-smelling orifice. Just be sure to never, ever purchase lubes that advertise "anal ease." Most lubes sold specifically for anal use contain large amounts of numbing agents, such as benzocane, which diminish sensation and will leave you with a numb tongue. They're manufactured by an industry that believes anal penetration of any kind is painful—when in reality, anal penetration isn't painful if you do it right. If it hurts, then something's wrong, and you don't want to mask important signals the body might be trying to send. Besides, who wants a numb butt?

Though rimming is certainly enjoyable, it isn't a very safe activity. Unprotected, it can transmit hepatitis A, anal herpes, anal warts, and possibly viruses such as HIV. Always use a barrier for rimming—but if you insist on barrier-free rimming, get a hepatitis A shot. If one of you has a viral STD, such as herpes, HPV, hepatitis C, or HIV, safer-sex practices are necessary—required—to prevent transmission, especially if you have a cut or bite in your mouth. Risk is greatly increased for both partners if you have recently brushed or flossed your teeth; both activities cause tiny cuts and bleeding in your mouth. For information on barriers for rimming and details on safersex practices , see chapter 4, "Know the Hard Facts: Health Considerations."

His Erotic Pressure Points

Touching your partner in specific areas while you're going down on him releases blocked sexual tension, increases his excitement and blood flow to the genital area, and can make orgasm much more powerful than usual. Several centuries ago, Chinese doctors concluded that certain points in the body held muscular tension that could accumulate and block the normal flow of circulation of energy. These acupuncture or acupressure points corresponded physically to medical ailments, and the doctors discovered that releasing tension through pressure on the blocked areas was medically therapeutic. They also discovered a range of erotic techniques.

Pressing acupressure points acts like a concentrated massage, releasing muscular tension and toxins held in the muscle, allowing blood and sensation to flow freely to the area. Increased circulation means increased feeling and responsiveness, which adds new dimensions of pleasure to fellatio.

You can activate pressure points by touching them in various ways—kissing, licking, caressing, sucking, kneading, and massaging—but the most effective way to employ them is to hold the point (or points) firmly with the pads of your fingers. Some points are more sensitive than others; you should avoid pressing directly on the high ridges of bones. Your nails should be short, and you should apply a gradual, slow, and direct pressure. If

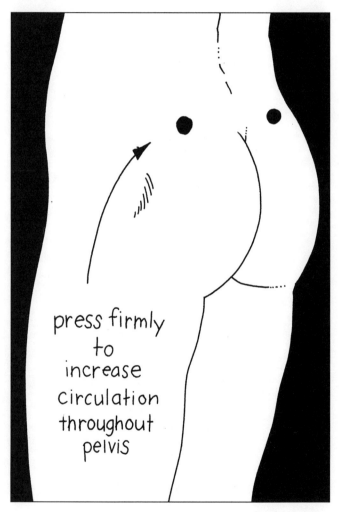

press firmly
to
increase
circulation
throughout
pelvis

Illustration #11. Increasing Circulation

the skin is pulling, lift up and reapply pressure directly to the point, as if you were pressing straight in. Hold each point for no more than five minutes at a time, and encourage him to breathe deeply as you press. Incorporate them at any stage during oral sex.

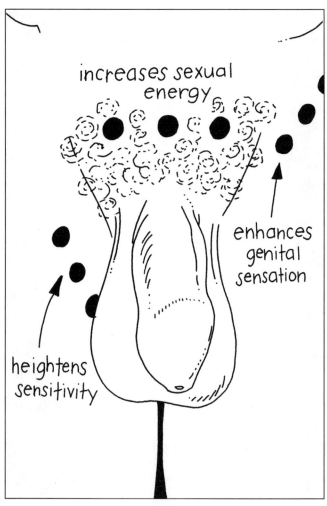

Illustration 12. Increasing Sexual Energy and Awareness

Increasing Sexual Energy and Awareness

Three points are located on the mons at the top edge of the pubic bone, in the center. Pressing them produces a warm, pleasant sensation and focuses energy and awareness on the entire genital system. This is great for helping him concentrate on arousal.

Enhancing Orgasm

You can apply pressure directly on the perineum to make orgasms more intense. This increases blood flow to the genital area and is beneficial to all reproductive and pleasure organs.

Heightening Sensitivity

On the inside of the upper thigh, right at the crease where the thigh meets the body in front, are six points that heighten pleasurable sensitivity and awareness. They amplify any genital pleasure you are providing.

Increasing Pleasure

These additional points on the base of the spine increase pleasure during oral sex and can be added to your erotic pressure point repertoire.

In general, applying pressure to his perineum or genital area with the flat of your hand or flattened fingertips feels great, because you're stimulating the entire system. You can also rub the mons while you suck, massage it in a circular motion, press it, or gently pull on it. Using genital massage techniques to begin or end a sexual activity, or to transition to another one, can turn a session of sex into a decadent encounter—use your imagination and these points as your guide.

Cough Drops and Ice Cubes

The sensations of heat and cold are remarkable in oral sex. Imagine a hot, wet mouth enveloping your genitals, licking and squeezing and radiating heat. Or a cool mouth caressing and rubbing you when you're so hot you're already at the melting point. That's the idea— using heat and coolness to prolong and increase arousal, or to turn up temperatures that are already in the triple digits.

You can bring temperature play into fellatio at any point when you want to tease or turn up the volume, though it's more effective in the earlier stages of sucking, before you get an orgasm-inducing rhythm going. There are two ways to go about it: applying the sensation to him directly, or changing the temperature of your mouth.

Direct Application

- Have a warm or cool washrag prepared in a bowl of warm or iced water at the bedside: pause your licking for a moment and apply the washrag, then continue. Make sure that a hot washrag isn't too hot, or it will burn—discreetly test it on the thin skin of your wrist first. If you're using an ice water compress, your tongue will feel hot and delicious on his cool cock.

- Set a bowl of ice cubes next to you, select one, and draw on his nipples, his stomach, and all over the area around his cock and balls.

- In warm water, have a number of items heated and ready: dildos, waterproof vibrators, washcloths. You can also pull a teabag out of a not-too-hot cup of tea and massage his cock or balls with it.

- In sex toy stores you can purchase lubricants that elicit hot or cool sensations and get more intense when you blow on them. These can be fun to play with, but they may not taste very good. Read more about them in chapter 4, "Know the Hard Facts: Health Considerations."

Changing the Temperature of Your Mouth

- From that bowl or cup of ice, put a cube in your mouth to cool down your tongue and lips.
- An iced or hot drink will change the temperature of your mouth perfectly—you'll know if it's too hot or cool because it will be uncomfortable for you, too. Pause while licking and take a mouthful of the beverage; swish and swirl it around your mouth for a minute, then swallow. Continue licking until you feel the temperature change, then repeat as necessary.

Cool and Tingling Sensations

When you pop a breath mint or a cough drop in your mouth, sometimes it feels like your entire oral cavity has the Arctic wind whistling through it—and that's not always an unpleasant feeling. Now, imagine that feeling on aroused genitalia, the coolness mixing with the arousing, enveloping wetness of your mouth. The feeling isn't for everyone—it can get pretty intense and feel too much like heat—but once some guys try it they like it a lot, so it's worth experimenting with to see if you can add it to your fellatio pleasure kit.

Menthol and mint cough drops and breath mints are amazing sex toys available next to practically every checkout counter in America. Try to find lozenges with both menthol and mint; they're the strongest. During oral play, put one (or two) in your mouth and swish it around to activate it and soften the corners—a sharp corner scraping his penis or the inside of your mouth would have you both thinking twice about trying it again. When you're good and mentholated, slip the lozenge between your cheek and gums. Putting it under your tongue will make it pop out, and trying to rest it on the back of your tongue while you lick could make you choke on it, so don't do either of those. The mentholated environment of your mouth will transfer the effects to his penis after just a minute, and you can also take the lozenge in your fingers and rub him with it, though you should avoid the urethral opening. You can also use mint and menthol on nipples, testicles, or the outside of the anus. Never insert anything into the anus that goes all the way in and disappears—even if you think it will dissolve. Add to the icy sensations by blowing softly on his penis and testicles.

The Flavored Penis

Chocolate or vanilla, darling? There are a lot of flavored lubes on the market that promise to turn any oral encounter into piña colada licks, tangerine sucks, or swallows of raspberry, cherry, or hazelnut. Flavored lubricants are readily available at any adult toy or novelty store, but the choice to use these sugary toppings is yours. They generally don't taste very good; imagine the flavor of lube mixed with artificial flavoring and sweetener. The pictures on the labels look much better than the products taste—and you may want to ask yourself what you do (or don't) want to be tasting, anyway. If the notion of oral sex is not appealing, then covering your lover's genitals with green kiwi goo isn't going to make the act feel any less distasteful. But if you just want to make the usual a little more unusual, or want to step out a little with a bit of playful accesorizing, then look before you shop and think about what you want to accomplish.

Edibles come in two categories: lubricants that are water-based and edible gels, liquids, or sprays that may contain oils. The distinction is important, because anything that contains oil will ruin latex. No matter how completely you think you are licking it off, even the smallest amount of oil can cause a condom, dental dam, or glove to break. Oils of any kind are difficult to flush out of the vagina, so if you think you might use whatever you flavored for penetration later, skip the oily stuff—that goes for whipped cream and chocolate, too.

Speaking of things going into vaginas, you'll want to think twice about what's in the flavored lube you use if vaginal penetration is on the menu. Oils are certainly on the list of things to avoid, but if you've got any sensitivities to yeast infections or your vaginal flora and fauna irritate easily, consider skipping the toppings altogether. The sugars and artificial colors/flavorings in edible lubes—and in other regular food items you might be inclined to use in oral play—can wreak havoc on the delicate balance of your vaginal ecosystem. If you want to use flavored lubes, honey, whipped cream, chocolate, or anything else that contains sugar, then save the penetration until after you scrub your sweetie clean in the shower.

Not to say that licking something yummy off of your lover isn't fun—it is. It can be a treat to have a little something extra to lick, something that makes your strokes longer and more focused. And adding blindfolds or restraints can really get things heated up. Imagine your pleasure victim all tied up, watching you pull out a strange container, and then you proceed to slather, and lick, and lick…The water-based brand ID Juicy Lube has by far the cleanest ingredient list, no artificial coloring, and the largest selection of flavors; I recommend sticking with their line of fruit flavors, though I admit Bubblegum Blast is pretty fun. Hot Licks is a super-sugary tasting line of water-based flavored gels that heat up when you breathe on them (though the heating-up sensation isn't for everyone), and they come in flavors like strawberry and cinnamon. Kama Sutra makes a whole range of products made for licking off excited body parts, and their Oil of Love also heats up; but keep in mind that many of their products contain trace amounts of oil.

To the Limit

A sex act of many masks, many hats, many costume changes, fellatio can slip seamlessly into as many scenarios as a seasoned actor. It's also wonderful to see how it slips in and out of a variety of guises within the context of realizing sexual fantasies, including gender play, role-play, power exchange, S/M, and bondage. You can use fellatio to enhance a fantasy, especially an edgy one, or vice-versa.

Using Fantasy in Reality

Sexual fantasy is the cornerstone of our individual sexual expression. An erotic fantasy is any thought, idea, image, or scenario that is sexually interesting to you. It doesn't have to be your number one turn-on, or it can be the one thing that gets your blood boiling. If you think you don't fantasize, think again. Fantasies can emerge from your erotic imagination in countless different forms, from fragmented to detailed. We all fantasize, whether in relation to sex or in other aspects of our lives. We may see famous people that are attractive and imagine that our lives overlap. We might revisit memories of times we have enjoyed, using them to make us feel good in the present. Often, we envision scenarios that have never happened and some that aren't even possible. Sometimes we tell others what we have actually done, fantasized about, or want to do, making a fantasy for them—or us—come true. Whatever shape your fantasies take, exploring them can open doors to understanding your arousal and can allow you to tap into new channels of erotic expression—channels that work for you.

It's important to keep in mind that fantasies don't necessarily bear any relationship to reality. The realm of fantasy is the sanctuary in your mind where you are free to enjoy things that you would never do in real life. And fantasy is not only where we can court the forbidden; it is also a powerful sex toy that can be used for arousal, heightening pleasure, and achieving climax.

Think about your fantasies for a moment, whether they are vivid, vague, seemingly mundane, or a little scary. Don't try to look deeply into their meanings, just pick out their main themes. What you're doing is isolating what it is that makes them a peak erotic experience for you. Keep your mind open, and don't pass judgment on yourself—this isn't about "good" and "bad," it's about understanding what turns you on. Note what stands out, and the important differences between what is possible in fantasy and what is possible in reality.

Think about what your favorite themes are, or try on new ideas that appeal to you. Try to feel comfortable with tapping into what these fantasies trigger when you want to become aroused. Remember that if you fanta-size about something shocking, like being forced to

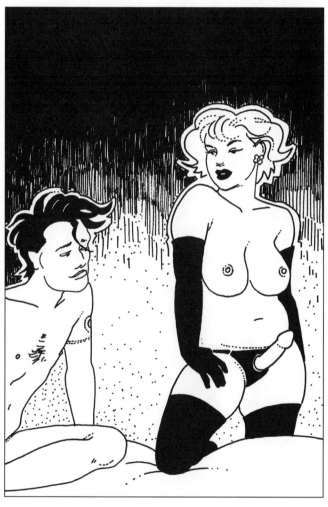

Illustration 13. Strap-On

perform sex, it doesn't mean that you want this to happen or that you are a bad person. But by identifying it in the realm of your fantasies, you can find a safe space where imagination fuels desire. By learning how to turn yourself on with fantasy, you can do extraordinary things—for instance, you can make yourself really aroused and teach yourself a new masturbation technique. Or you can fantasize while you go down on your partner, and turn yourself on with the combination of stimuli; the reverse works when your lover fantasizes as you go down on him. Or if you have established trust and sexual communication with your lover, you can share your fantasies—you can even make some of them come true.

Once you know what your favorite fantasy elements are, you can take steps to use them in fantasy scenarios that you cook up with your partner. Here are some ideas for inspiration:

- Firsts: you experience a first time engaging in a sexual act such as penetration, oral sex, or anal sex.
- Loss of control: someone has sexual power over you, "makes" you do things.
- Having control: you exert sexual power, have people "service" you.
- Taboo: you have sex with a forbidden person such as a clergyman or family member, an animal, or someone of the same gender. You can also incorporate inappropriate urges or timing, or even rape.
- Multiple partners: you experience a gang-bang, sex with the football team, a sex party, an orgy, a threesome.
- Casual or anonymous partners: you have sex with strangers, a waitress, the UPS guy.

- Your partner: you relive a memory of them, they engage in different behavior such as dominance or submission, or you have a peak experience with them.
- Public spaces: you have sex in the office, movie theater, park, dressing room.
- Being "used": you are a slave or a fuck toy, or get passed around among many people.
- Role-play: you and/or your partner can be an icon, such as a cop, schoolgirl, hooker, doctor, nurse, dog, dog owner.
- Romance: you can imagine yourself in dreamy situations, such as being seduced by a rock star or actor, or making love tenderly to the girl at the office.
- Objectification/fetish: you can focus on anything— breasts, butts, dicks, mouths, panties, shoes...
- Gender play: you trade genders, one of you is a different gender, he becomes a woman you're going down on, you become a gay man who "cruises" him.

Tips for Fellatio Threesomes

Adding a friend to an oral sex encounter can be fun. Be sure that you and your lover (or the partners you are joining) genuinely feel comfortable mixing sex with the relationships involved. It's highly recommended that you all talk before you get down to business. State your intentions clearly. Discuss your expectations—find out who just wants to have fun and if anyone sees the experience as a way of deepening a relationship. Ask if anyone might be jealous for any reason, and tell everyone that they can stop the action at any point if they feel weird or uncomfortable, and that it's okay. If you don't get a chance to talk about it—because these things sometimes just happen—make sure you're okay with what's going on, and if it's your first time, see it as an experiment that you can walk away from, mystery solved. And do it for you—because it turns you on, or because it makes you hot to fulfill your lover's fantasy.

Here are some ideas about what you might do in a threesome:

- Team up with a friend to go down on him. Take turns with his cock, passing it back and forth like a treat.
- Have your friend jack him off into your mouth. Try jacking him off into your friend's mouth.
- Lick his balls, perineum, or ass while your friend fellates him, or vice-versa.
- Fuck him with a strap-on while the other person fellates him.
- Have someone go down on (or penetrate) you while you suck him off, or vice-versa.
- Sit on his face while the other person gives him head, or turn around while you are giving him head and have your friend lick you in a "daisy chain."
- Play around with roles and control. Both of you can order him around, tell him he's your love slave or suck toy. You can order your friend to suck him, or reverse roles, and so on. He could be the one in charge, with both of you his oral sex slaves. Have fun!

Tips for Public Fellatio

She sat me down in this big blue chair in the room. She faced the chair toward the computer, so the back was facing the door and blocking it a little. She crawled under the desk. She quickly undid my shorts and boxers. She started giving me an incredible blow job. It was fucking amazing. At one point, somebody even knocked on the door and opened it. She stopped. I turned a little. I was asked a question, quickly gave an answer, the guy never came inside the room, and she continued to give me, without question, the best head ever.

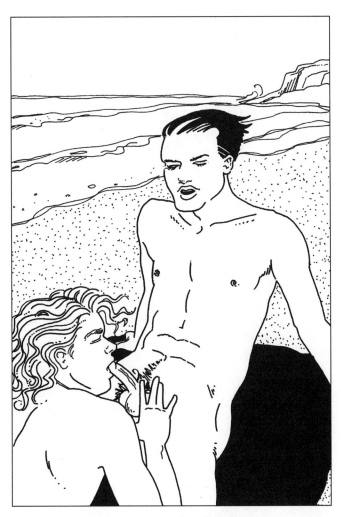

Illustration 14. Fellatio at the Beach

Fellatio can happen virtually anywhere, and the sexual tension that stems from possible discovery is what gives a public encounter its heat. Just remember that when someone sees you having sex in public, not only is it illegal, but you are essentially forcing someone to watch a sex act—they don't have any choice, even if it's an accident. So don't throw caution totally to the wind and involve someone without their consent in your steamy fantasy-come-true: think it through and get away with it, clean! Visit the spot you have in mind before you attempt a sexual encounter. Make sure you know the area well enough that you can avoid being seen, or avoid any possible dangers.

- Seek out reliably secluded spots, such as a remote place to park the car, a deserted beach, a vacant warehouse, an empty movie theater.
- Some places in large cities are notorious for being public sex spots. Use these places only if you are a local and are familiar with the area. If you must cruise, proceed with streetwise caution.
- Rooftops can seem public but still be private. Look around first, before you're horny.
- If you plan on using safer-sex gear, make sure you have it in your pocket.
- Think ahead about places to duck for cover, ways to camouflage your activity, or a story to tell a possible authority figure.
- Make it as hot and fun as you can—public fellatio is a thrilling encounter that can never be exactly duplicated. Don't hold back.

Power Exchange

You can add an extra dimension to oral sex when you play around with power balance, or rather, power imbalance. When you both arrive to the sexual table on equal footing in terms of who is in control, it can be an exchange on very pleasant and pleasurable terms. But when someone has a little—or a lot more—of the upper hand, make sure your perishables are refrigerated, because it's a sure bet that temperature will rise.

Power exchange and fellatio can come in a variety of flavors. First, the power tipping can come from either side of the fellatio equation. The person getting head can be the one in control, "using" the mouth (and any other part he likes) to achieve his satisfaction. Conversely, the person giving him head can be the one calling the shots, "making" him submit to any whim, pain, or pleasure you choose to dole out. He has to do what you say to get what he wants, and you don't have to let him come until you're satisfied.

> She sat there for a second with my cock in her mouth, then began moving up and down on it just a tiny bit. I put my hand on the back of her head, wanting to move it up and down more, wanting to fuck her mouth, and she slapped it down. Instead, she just kept her mouth there, barely moving it…

Your fellatio power play can be subtle, sneaky, extreme—anything that turns you both on. It can be as easy as giving him a knowing look, a push back against a wall to say "I'm in control," and then making your way downward. You can be a little more quick and forceful, especially in a public or semipublic place (like a car), pushing and pulling him whichever way you want him. Blindfold him and you're in total control. In the exchange of power, the reverse can be just as fun; he can be the one pushing, pulling, commanding you to suck, swallow. And your scenes can become more carefully orchestrated, planned with roles, sex toys, or costumes—or all three. Let your fantasies guide you.

Gender Play

Just as tipping the scales of power can be fun with fellatio, so can playing around with the boundaries of gender. I like to think of what we've got when we're born (in terms of gender) as the medium we have to work with; however we want to bend it to our pleasure and to fit our fantasies is all part of the fun of sex and sexual fantasy. Having or even acting out opposite-gender fantasies can be titillating as all get-out, but these fantasies don't change our identity. If it turns you on, it's a great way to get off, but it doesn't mean that you're a different person or that you don't like who you are—actually, it's a signifier that you're very secure with who you are, so secure that you can articulate your fantasies and desires.

Gender play can also be used to help flesh out emerging identities. Someone who knows that they are transgender might find that gender play in sex reinforces who they really feel themselves to be, whether through fantasy or with sex toys. A transgender woman could find that she really feels good and gets off when she fantasizes that her cock being sucked is her pussy being licked; a man in a woman's body can be sent over the edge into orgasm when his clit is fellated as if it were his cock.

Straight, bi, lesbian, gay male, and trans couples get a lot of mileage out of gender swapping in fellatio. Straight folks have reinvented sex with the overwhelmingly popular recent addition of the strap-on to their frolics. Not only are women enjoying penetrating men with their silicone dicks, but we're also discovering how hot it is to get our new cocks sucked by our boyfriends—and they're finding that it drives them wild. Lesbians and dykes have been bending gender along the fellatio continuum for a while now, role-playing as dykes with dicks, straight couples, or even pairs of gay men.

When a Little Pain Is Nice

You've probably heard people refer to things that "feel so good they almost hurt," and the phrase "hurts so good" has managed to linger in our collective consciousness for, well, since I was a kid. That's because the concepts of pleasure and pain are like twin pups in the human catalog of emotion and sensation; they're separate animals but often like to play together. In sex, the pleasure and pain lines mingle often, and in ways we aren't always aware of. Grabbing and squeezing your lover can easily give way to pulling, pinching, biting, and scratching—in small portions or stronger doses, depending on urge and response. The stronger the urge to, say, pull hair, and the more erotic and pleasurable the response, the more force will be applied. We humans love to up the ante in sex, and when we're blissed out on hormones, endorphins, and lust, we can easily add a little pleasurable pain to the mix.

Squeezing his thighs or ass a little harder than usual when you're giving him a blow job isn't out of the ordinary, but if you're planning on doing much more than that you'll need to learn about what you're doing, and make sure it's okay before you proceed. Intense sensations during sex are to be negotiated beforehand. Consult chapter 1, "More Than a Mouthful," about talking to your lover, and reference the book suggestions in chapter 12, "Independent Study," for further guidance.

The threshold of mingling pleasure with pain can be crossed in a variety of guises. The two of you may have decided that that you want to add pain into fellatio as if it were a sex toy, and simply experiment with techniques and toys. Or, it could be that you have a fantasy scenario in mind in which one of you is dominant and the other submissive, and some spanking or rough play fuels the fantasy's fire. You could be a teacher, and he the naughty pupil who gets a spanking and then some oral sex. Perhaps you just want to play the dominant woman or man, and take rough surveys of his nipples, cock, and balls as you fellate him. He may simply enjoy the way pain adds to the feeling of getting head; or perhaps one particular thing pushes him over the edge, such as nipple biting upon orgasm, and role-play or fantasy don't enter into it at all. Pain, as a sex toy, can be shaped to fit your own personal sex style.

> My girlfriend and I sometimes like to play rough, where I overpower and dominate her in various ways. One thing we both like is when I grab her in the hallway or someplace, and push her down to her knees, and hold her hair tightly as I push my penis into her mouth. She knows I won't push farther than she can take, but she also likes the feeling of being mock-forced to suck me.

You have several options literally at your fingertips when you want to increase the pleasure/pain volume during fellatio. You have the choice of breaking from the action and doing things to other parts of his body, such as lightly spanking his thighs or ass, or you can suck and give him little bites on his ass, stomach, chest, or nipples. Some men really enjoy having their nipples roughly stimulated when they're close to orgasm. You can scratch him with your fingernails anywhere that's pleasurable, but refrain from ticklish areas unless he's one of those rare guys who get off on being tickled. When administering pain, and blending it with pleasure, be sure to give him almost what he wants, then back off and make him want it, bad. Don't go for the intense sensations right away; go lighter than he wants, then give him a little more.

His penis can be given little bits of painful stimulation that you can alternate with pleasurable cocksucking techniques. Some men like just a little pain here and there on their penis; a few may like continuous pain. His cock can be squeezed with your hand and sucked roughly, and the skin can be pinched or pulled. If you know it's okay with him, you can play around with your teeth on his penis, lightly running them around the head or along the shaft. Some men enjoy having their penis spanked lightly, but don't miss and hit his balls—unless you know explicitly that this is okay with him. Cup his cock in your hand or have it pointed upward, flat on his stomach. His balls are right there, waiting to be squeezed, pulled, pinched, or constricted. Never slap or spank his testicles, or constrict them with too much pressure or force, or it will become the wrong kind of pain, the pain that stops the fellatio. Watch his nonverbal reactions, or check in with him by asking specific questions. Don't ask if something is "okay," because that word can mean anything. Ask if he wants it harder, softer, or tighter, if he wants more pinch or less movement, or if he wants you to stop.

Pausing from the blow job, you can apply clamps or clips to his body parts, or specifically his penis and testicles, to elicit a low-level, continuous hum of pain as you give him head. Apply clips to any area where you can pinch enough skin for the clamp—use common sense and don't try to put a clamp on a flat area or an area where it's difficult to get some skin between your fingers. Clamps and clips deliver concentrated pinching sensations to the body part they're applied to, and they pinch at first, then turn into a steady buzz of pain; then, when you take them off, sensation rushes to the area and there's a burst of intense pain. Get to know the pain cycle of clips by trying one on yourself, in a sensitive area like the inside of your arm, and you'll see that while they hurt going on, they hurt much more coming off. You can use this knowledge to time the sensations with your oral overtures, or with his pleasure cycle.

Little clamps can be purchased practically anywhere, from an S/M boutique to a stationery store. Clamps and clips made specifically for S/M play are best for sex. These have already been designed for sexual purposes, taking into consideration that they might be going onto sensitive areas or thin skin. Small clips are usually plastic with a spring that you pinch open, though you can also find metal versions. Even though a clip may be small, it can be pretty mean, because it concentrates the pain in one small area. Medium to large clips can be plastic or metal, even similar to the clips you'd use to keep a bag of potato chips fresh. Make sure that the ends of any metal clamps are padded or encased in rubber, and that any clips you use do not have teeth.

Wooden, plastic, and specialty metal clothespins fall into the "mean" category. Clothespins are intense. Be sure to always test each clothespin before you use it, as they have differing intensities depending on how tight the spring is. You can lessen the pinch by forcing the spring open slightly with a pair of pliers. Nipple clamps often have a way to adjust the pressure, such as a slide ring on tweezers, or a tightening screw on alligator clamps. These are fun because you can vary the pressure on whatever part of him you have clamped—for instance, you can increase pressure by tiny increments as arousal increases. Limit the time you keep the clip on; you should take them off after fifteen to thirty minutes to avoid tissue damage.

Pain, Pain, Don't Go Away

Should you find that you and the man you're going down on really like playing with pain during fellatio, that it really turns you both on and increases his pleasure, arousal, and orgasm, there are plenty of ways to safely push the pain a little further. Cock and ball play—or CBT, cock and ball torture—can be intensely pleasurable to a man who enjoys erotic pain in the sensitive, nerve-rich area of his genitals. It can be in any context: punishment, humiliation, reward, torture, a meaningful ordeal or ritual, or just part of hot sex. You should first discuss any type of sex play in which you will be inflicting pain on his genitals. Be absolutely clear about what is "good" pain to him and what constitutes "bad" pain. Find out what he likes about it; ask specific questions, and make sure to agree on specific thing that he wants you to do to him. This is called *negotiation*—you're negotiating desires, activities, and most important, limits. Decide on a *safe word*—a word that he will say when he absolutely wants you to stop.

There are different ways you can administer pain, and you can vary the levels of pain as well. Types of stimulation include friction, pressure, pinching, slapping, constriction, spanking, flogging, piercing, and more—and you can use these in a plethora of ways. Your spanks on his penis or buttocks can get harder, faster, stingier. You might bring in a toy like a leather or rubber slapper and alternate sucking and spanking. You can lightly whip his balls with a small flogger, and you can whip his penis even harder. Small floggers will help you avoid injury to his testicles; you can use larger (medium-sized) ones on his penis. Your bites can linger longer, press a little harder (but no breaking the skin, please). Pinches on nipples can seem endless, or they can come off with a twist—and so can clamps.

Clips and clamps can be played like piano keys with your fingers—and the sounds he makes might be music to your ears, even if they are not on key. When the clips are on and you're fellating him, you can give him bursts of pain (reminding him that the clips are there) by simply touching them, pulling on the surrounding skin, or flicking them with your fingers. Pulling and twisting hurts even more. If you put clips on his penis or testicles, you don't have to avoid them during your blow job; lick and suck on the clips, or fellate his cock, clips and all. You can wrap rubber bands around larger clips to make them tighter or to pull several together. Lay a piece of thin cotton or nylon rope under a row of clips, and pull on one end of the rope as you would on a zipper, removing the clips slowly or in one blindingly painful zip. You can also rig ropes and clips to small fishing weights, available where fishing supplies are sold.

You can use a pinwheel, the device doctors use to determine nerve response, everywhere except his penis, testicles, and anal opening. This sinister-looking and very painful medical instrument consists of an 8-inch handle, with a small stainless steel rolling wheel at one end that has very sharp pin pricks. When the wheel is rolled lightly over skin, it leaves a trail of sharp pain and a fiery sensation in its wake. This dastardly device is handy for use during fellatio, but be sure to have half your mind on his cock and the other half on the wheel, making sure you roll it lightly to avoid piercing the skin too deeply. And don't share your pinwheel with other partners, unless you have access to hospital sterilization.

Cock rings shouldn't hurt when they're on, but they can be made to, and you can find ones that are made for pain rather than constriction. Rings can be tightened, or layered one on top of the other to up the ante. Some cock rings have steel D-rings on them, allowing you to attach a fishing weight or a leash; fishing weights should be gently lowered with your hand, and leashes should never be yanked on. Ball stretchers, cock and ball vises, ball stocks, ball separators, and combination cock ring/ball "torture" devices can all be found at specialty S/M boutiques, especially ones that cater to gay men. These toys will bring out the Inquisitor in you, and ideally the delighted moans of pleasurable pain from him, but they should be used only by experienced players. Consult the book recommendations in chapter 12, "Independent Study," for books that explain safe exploration of CBT.

Tie Me Up, Tie Me Down: Bondage

Using restraint during oral sex can heighten the tension of your session, literally! Whether you're into bondage or not, rope, handcuffs, leather cuffs, or anything you use to restrain someone can immobilize arms, legs, or an entire body while fellatio is being performed. Some people like the physical feeling of being tied up more than anything, and find that straining against ropes or struggling to move their arms or legs when they are about to explode sends them through the roof. Having one of you tied up can enhance one partner's sense of helplessness—or the other one's feeling of power. He might find that having his cock sucked when you're in total physical control of him makes his orgasms more powerful, and he might enjoy playing victim to your inner sexual predator. Or, you may enjoy being tied up yourself, while he "makes" you please him orally. Either partner might find that their arousal is enhanced by being restrained.

In other parts of this book I've touched briefly on master/slave and dominant/submissive contexts for fellatio, and the unique ability of oral sex to slip into many molds, many scenarios. When the receiver is dominant, ordering his partner to give him head strengthens his role as a master or top. And the reverse may be equally true: when you go down on him, it might be a pleasure you dole out as a dominant, a reward for good behavior, or to prolong erotic torture in which you never give him enough of what he needs. He may relish the feeling of being able to relax and let you take over, or in reverse, his controlling your mouth and telling you what to do may be the type of "letting go" that gets you off. This type of role-play takes fellatio to another level, deepening the experience with a mixture of power and devotion.

Don't confine your efforts to controlling his limbs; investigate the world of possibilities afforded by sight restriction. So simple, yet so effective, a blindfold can be used on its own or in combination with any of the other techniques in this book to create an oral sex experience he won't forget. A blindfold takes away his sight, making him depend on you more for sensory information, heightening his awareness of his physicality, making him helpless and hyperaware at the same time. Because he can't see what you're up to, it gives you extra room to relax, knowing that he's both unsteady and unable to watch you.

Take my advice and buy an actual blindfold. Don't bother with scarves, ties, or silky undergarments, even when improvisation might be sexy. Blindfolds made specifically for sex fit better and more comfortably, and they restrict sight more reliably. Many are padded or have fake fur inside, and have wide elastic straps or are adjustable for the comfort of the wearer. Improvised items may become painfully tight or uncomfortable, or loosen and slip, coming off at inopportune moments. Plus, you don't want to be worrying about the blindfold when you're concentrating on his cock, and you don't want him left with blurry vision or a headache—you want him hungry for more of what you're giving him.

Men at Work

by Alison Tyler

Maybe there's no such thing as love at first sight, but lust at first sight...well, that's a different story altogether. Because that's what I had, and I had it bad. Lust for the dark-haired, dark-eyed captain of a rough-and-rowdy road crew.

The crew had been out in our little rural community for weeks. Trimming trees. Moving boulders. And making me want to come. Not all of them. Just one of them. A fiercely handsome man with a sleek mustache and sparkling brown eyes. He'd look at me when he was the one holding up the Stop sign, and I'd look back through the windshield, flush, and look away. How many times? Three, four—every fucking time I went to do an errand. And I went to do more errands than usual when I knew they were at work. I put on elaborate make-up just to go to the grocery store. Normally a jeans-and-T-shirt-type of girl, I wore skirts and high-heeled leather boots, and I took extra time styling my long black hair.

After several weeks of visual foreplay, I got bold. I held his eye contact and stared back at him, gazed through my cherry-flush, forcing the connection. He liked that. He tilted his head at me and narrowed his eyes, and I could almost hear what he was thinking. Take me on? Is that what you think you're doing, little girl? You think you can take me?

The men were connected to one another with walkie-talkies, alerting each other when cars were waiting at either end of the road work. One afternoon, I watched a heavy-set man radio another while the Stop sign was in place. After a moment, he flipped the sign to Slow and motioned me forward. As I drove around the windy roads, I spotted a golden-yellow work truck in my rear-view mirror. Was it him? How was I supposed to find out?

I kept on my normal route, I saw the truck holding steady, and finally I pulled into the dirt lot of a local park. Empty. Totally empty. Surrounded by trees. Hidden. The truck pulled in behind me, and my man got out. I knew in my head what I wanted to do, but I didn't know whether people really behaved like that outside of porno movies. Could I step from my convertible, rush over, and tell him what to do to me? Turned out I didn't have to. He knew. True doms can always sniff out a sub.

With a nod of his head, he motioned for me to come toward him. I slid from my seat, slammed the door behind me, and walked to the back of his truck. As soon as I was in his range, he gripped onto my shoulders and brought me into his arms for a kiss—the kiss I'd imagined since I'd first seen him. Hot and fast, his mouth firm against mine, his teeth finding my bottom lip and then biting it hard. Then, because it had to happen, because it was right, he pushed me down on the gravel-strewn dirt and unbuttoned his deeply faded jeans. I was ready, my lips parted, mouth open, but he stopped me before I could act. Quickly, he pulled his heavy leather belt free from his jeans, and with me in the exact position he wanted, he captured my wrists tightly behind my back.

"Such a tease," he said, running his fingers roughly under my chin, tilting my head upward with a jerk. "Such a fucking tease."

I sighed, so hungry now, so desperate, but he wasn't ready to give in. All I wanted was the taste of his cock in my mouth, and I wanted it more than anything I've ever craved, yet he wouldn't let me suckle him. With one hand still under my chin, he ran the back of his free hand against my cheek, softly, making me tremble all over at the gentleness of his touch. Then his hand came up high in the air, and he slapped my cheek, catching me off-guard, making me bite down on a moan. I lowered my head, shuddering all over, feeling how wet my panties were growing. Feeling how much I needed this. Needed him to treat me exactly the way he was.

"Look at me, baby," he insisted, and I raised my head.

Now, he pushed forward, butting against my lips with the head of his cock. Oh, God, oh Christ, was I ready. I wanted to drink, wanted to drain, wanted to swallow him whole. But still he wouldn't let me. He plunged in, taking his pleasure, then slid back out and bent to rub my nipples forcefully through my thin white blouse. He pinched them hard, and I arched and groaned, and while my mouth was open, he slid his cock in again. Each time he played me, he made me wetter still. So that I didn't know what I was doing anymore. All I knew was I had the need—the urgency—to drink him down.

"Bad girl," he said, "lost in your little games. Cruising the curves in your silver convertible. And all you want is for someone to fuck that sweet mouth of yours. Isn't that right?"

I think I nodded. I know I moaned. And he let me, finally, let me have at him. I swallowed with a vengeance. I sucked and pulled, my cheeks indenting with the intensity of my hunger. He held me steady with his rough hands on my shoulders, pinned me in place in his strong grip. My eyes wide open, I saw the trees behind him, saw his scuffed work boots below, the dirt under my knees. It was a relief to be allowed to use my mouth, to trick my tongue up and down his straining rod. I almost cried with the release of tasting the first drops of his pre-come.

When I could think of nothing more than draining his every drop, he pulled out again, lifted me up by my arms, and bent me over. Holding me steady, my skirt captured up at my waist, he slid my panties all the way down my legs and waited for me to step out of them. Then he punished my naked ass with his large open hand, spanking me hard and fast. All my faith was in him. He had the total control to keep me balanced, so that I wouldn't fall forward against the gravel, so that I wouldn't collapse on the ground. I had no thoughts now; I simply let him take me. Let him push me back down again onto the scraped raw skin of my knees, so that I could open my mouth wide and suck him. Sweetly suck him. My mouth earning the pleasure of the power he imparted.

Up and down my tongue tricked against his shaft. In and out his cock plunged, searching out the warm, wet heat of my throat. I was delirious with the pleasure of serving him. Breathing deeply, I memorized his smell, the way his skin felt against my cheeks, the way my ass smarted under the gauzy fabric of my summer-weight skirt. Then he was once again in motion, lifting me up and bringing me to the back of the truck. My wrists were still bound behind my back, so he had to slide my skirt up for me, kicking my legs wider apart, pushing into me with the spit-slicked length of his erection. He fucked me so hard that his truck shook. My face pressed into the metal of the truck bed; my honeyed juices spilled down my thighs. And when we were finished, he simply unbuckled the well-worn belt and set me free.

But I didn't want to be free.

"You're calmer now, aren't you, girl?"

I thought about the words before I answered, and then I nodded. He was right. All the nervous energy that had pulsed through me each time we'd made eye contact was now gone. I felt warm and in control. Better yet, I felt satisfied. I watched him get into the truck and drive out of the lot.

I don't know when the road crew will be back, but I do know that I'll be ready.

Independent Study: Erotic Videos and Books

Erotic videos and books are a goldmine for inspiration, education, and titillation. Explicit adult fiction can transport you into fantasies that can turn you on, or you can read aloud to your partner to turn them on; you can even take turns reading to each other as you go down on each other. Get a good sex guidebook and you can supplement the information you already know, take any desires you discovered in this book even further, or get a conversation going with your lover. Adult videos can be used like sex toys, too: watch some hot head in action and you might blow your top, or you can watch it together and imitate the actors onscreen. I'm going to recommend many different videos and books, and while not all of them will be to your individual liking, they're the best that's out there and are reliably hot. All of my choices are explicit; you won't find any soft-focus approaches to sex in the following sections. Consider your preferences, and look at the suggestions to see what tickles your fancy.

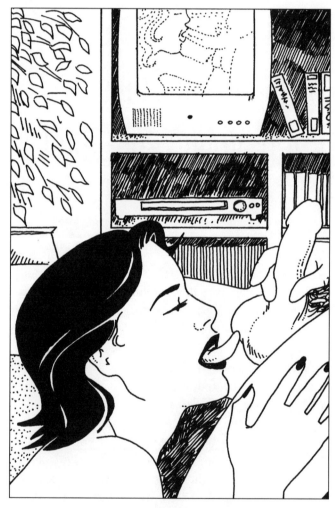

Illustration 15. A Little Inspiration

How to Watch Erotic Videos

I used to be turned off by the type of porn where the girl holds her mouth open and the guy comes into it, but it became so dirty for me that oddly enough, now it's my biggest turn-on.

Everyone's got a different take on adult movies, and these perspectives generally boil down to two views: either you consider these films offensive, or you see using the explicit imagery the same way you'd use a sex toy—to get off. As you can probably tell, I'm in the latter category. But all porn isn't created equal, and there's a lot of lame, poor-quality, and quite offensive stuff out there—though as we know from watching the legal wranglings of the art world in the United States, obscenity and offensiveness are in the eye of the beholder. If you want to steer clear of specific sex acts or other things you might not like, then you might want to do a little reading here before you do a little watching at home.

If you're thinking about renting or buying a blue move, then you're not alone. According to the Free Speech Coalition's 1999 survey of adult retailers, during 1998 stores in the United States reported a total of 686 million rentals of adult tapes. Typically when we think of the people who rent these videos, we think of the stereotype of men in raincoats—and while that might fit part of the population, these guys are practically extinct today. It's certainly true that the average viewer is male, but the viewership has changed dramatically over the last twenty-five years to include more women and couples of all orientations.

If you're a woman reading this, it's possible that admitting to yourself that you want to watch porn is confusing or difficult. One of the major obstacles that we women face is the widely held notion that women don't respond to sexual imagery the way men do—which is absolutely untrue. In her 1994 study, Dr. Ellen Laan of the University of Amsterdam found that women responded physiologically to sexual images, even when the women said that the porn they watched was boring or unarousing. When the women in the study watched the sex onscreen (whether from male or female directors), their genitals congested with blood, proving they were having a sexual response.

Once you feel okay about using porn as a sex toy, there are a few things you need to know before you get started. First, keep your expectations in check—you're not going to see films the quality of mega-budget Hollywood blockbusters. Why not? Because outside of Hollywood studios, no one has that kind of money or resources to throw around, especially in a film genre that's controversial.

The quality you are going to see is that of daytime soap operas: simple sets, standard lighting, digital cameras, and barely-there acting. Unless you go with a film from a bigger studio; the world of porn has a studio system just like in Hollywood. The big studios (like Vivid and VCA) have bigger budgets, better sets, actors who might have gone to acting school, writers with writing experience, and directors who are more likely to take their craft seriously, some even using real film stock in their movies.

Just as with any other sex toy, it helps if you're aroused before you begin watching porn. When you put the tape in and press Play, be sure to have the following items ready: lube, a dildo, vibrator, and towel, and the remote control. Having a sex toy ready if you need it is handy, because if the video turns you on and you want to get off, you won't have to interrupt the moment to search for your toys.

But why the remote control? The remote is the only really required item for porn viewing: you'll need to fast-forward through anything you don't like, or whatever distracts you from your arousal—be it lame dialogue, a sex act you don't prefer, or an unsightly boob job. For some people this may seem like a hassle at first—why can't they just make the "perfect" porno?

The makers of porn try to appeal to as many tastes as possible in a relatively short amount of time. Porn has to get to the point pretty quickly in order to retain horny viewers who usually want instant gratification, and so, like Hollywood, they've boiled down what they think viewers want into formulas. These are typical-male type formulas—that is, typical males of about twenty years ago.

The formulas include six to seven sex scenes, a standard set of positions and couplings, actors and actresses with mostly shaved genitals, men with larger-than-normal penises, and women with larger-than-normal breasts—with a few notable exceptions. An oft-voiced complaint is that the men are acceptable when unlovely in fitness and form, while the women's bodies must conform to a standard: underweight, blonde hair, big lips, and big boobs (the Beverly Hills Plastic Surgery Association is always well represented). Almost always, the men pull out before orgasm and ejaculate on the other person's face, breasts, ass, or vulva, so the viewer can see it. To say the least, little emphasis is placed on female orgasm and ejaculation—but that's changing in the industry as we speak.

Think about what expectations you're bringing to your adult video. This will help you make a selection that won't leave you high and dry, or in the worst-case scenario, angry at the genre. What ideas turn you on— small breasts, big butts, women in charge, realistic plots, blow jobs, two gals and a guy, male anal penetration, group sex? This may not be your list, but you get the idea. Get clear on what you want to avoid by making another list of things you don't want to see—do you get turned off by fake breasts, hairy men, rimming, toe sucking, facial ejaculation, two women together, or anal sex? These are just examples to get you brainstorming about what you'll want to look for, and what you'll want to fast-forward through. You may find more to add to either list as you view tapes—sometimes we find things that turn us on or off that we didn't even know about.

Knowing what you like and dislike can help enormously when selecting a tape. You can single out many of your preferences before you rent or buy, and then skip the parts you don't care for. The reviews on Web sites of women-run sex toy stores are very helpful in these matters—I should know, because I've been writing these reviews for years. The reviews and ratings can also help you select videos that include things you don't usually see on the blue screen, such as an all-natural cast (enhancement-free), internal ejaculation, attention to cinematography and lighting, great acting, and excellent plots.

There are certain things in porn that are hard to avoid even if you don't like them. Facial ejaculation (the man ejaculating on his sex partner's face) is pretty much a standard. So are boob jobs. I hear a lot of complaints about both of these things, but some people, somewhere, like them. If you want to avoid "facials" in straight porn, look for porn made by women directors such as Veronica Hart and Candida Royalle. Both women make excellent plot-driven movies, and if you want to avoid anal sex, Candida rarely features it in her films. Finding all-natural starlets is a little tricky, but there are more of them now than five years ago. Look for porn made by independent movie companies.

Fellatio in porn is largely performed for the camera's view, and what the director thinks the viewers want to see—not for either performer's enjoyment. Typically, the person going down will have their face angled in a way that is not very comfortable or practical for giving head in real life. This is because the camera and lights have to get close to the action, and if it's a woman with long hair, her head needs to be cocked at an angle that keeps her mane flowing down the opposite side of her head. The techniques the actors use are basic but can be learned from somewhat, if only to see how they use their hand as an extension of their mouth or to stroke him while they back off for a brief rest. Porn is where you'll see a lot of deep throating and some amazing stamina on the part of both the giver and the receiver of the blow job. Don't expect to be able to duplicate what the actors can do—they're pros, and they give head for a living. Also, the scenes are not all shot in one take, and are often edited to make the scenes appear longer, or the activity more varied.

Watching fellatio in straight porn versus gay male porn, you'll notice a difference in enthusiasm, touch, and comfort with cock. The actors in gay male films know their way around a hard dick, most likely because they own one and understand the sensations they're delivering intimately. The gay actors usually appear less conscious of what they're doing and more relaxed; it's almost as if they didn't need to think about what they're doing. And a big overall difference is that the guys touch the other guys more than their female coun-terparts; the men's hands touch, squeeze, and roam all over the guys they go down on. But other than these points, there aren't a lot of differences, and there are certainly women in porn who have the same intuitive connection to and eagerness for the men they give head to onscreen.

Finding individual films can be challenging when there are hundreds of thousands cranked out in a given year. Also, many adult retailers don't carry every title, not to mention that selection and organization in sex shops can be haphazard. So I'm not going to recom-mend films; instead, I'm going to give you the names of actors who give drop-dead head and whose enthusiasm for sucking cock will make you weak in the knees. In straight porn, certain women do it right and just can't get enough: look for Chloe, Jeanna Fine, Linda Lovelace, Missy, Juli Ashton, and Nina Hartley.

How-To Videos

Educational videos can give you great visual references for techniques, though sadly many are dated, or just look dated. Many oral sex instructional videos, new or old, are shot the same ways and have a timeless quality that unfortunately hovers around the 1980s: fireplace and fur rug sets, women wearing pearls and big jewelry, fluffy hair on both genders, talking heads perched on chairs explaining everything—"experts" intended to make you feel comfortable and nonsleazy, though this has the opposite effect on me. Much like with the fella-tio guidebook counterparts, it's pretty slim pickings—for now. At this time, there are no how-to instructional oral sex films that are same-sex oriented; they're all straight.

But many of the films feature real-life couples, and they almost always use natural-bodied actors.

Adult how-to videos are explicit and often contain extra noninstructional sex scenes that make them worth your money. These videos come in two flavors: mainstream adult films made by porn stars or films independently produced by individuals, sex toy companies, or sex organizations. The mainstream films are usually missing some component of accuracy and are packed with porn stars giving eager, though sometimes mechanical, demonstrations. The independents make up for what they lack in budgets and the actors' on-camera presence by featuring normal folks, usually real-life, clearly loving couples.

In the realm of fellatio, there are a couple tapes that can show you how to do some of the things discussed in this book and can provide sexy inspiration. *Nina Hartley's Making Love to Men* is one part information, several parts explicit action—and parts of it are quite arousing to watch. It's Nina's most recent and her best tape on the subject. *Better Oral Sex Techniques* is a Sinclair Institute video, part of their series of how-to tapes, and like all Sinclair tapes, it features actual couples. However, the sex is broken up by more talking heads, and the video presents the information in an annoying numbered sequence. The *Complete Guide to Oral Lovemaking* has a 1980s feel to it (hair and lingerie, especially) and is full of talking heads. Its information is straightforward, but don't expect any in-depth descriptions of fellatio, or advanced techniques.

How-to tapes about male sexuality are rare, but there are a few that can enrich and complement a healthy sex life. Joseph Kramer has done some wonderful video work, and you can learn through his spiritual approach how to give a man a great erotic massage in *Fire on the Mountain: An Intimate Guide to Male Genital Massage*. The tone is quite New Age, but the video presents great techniques and excellent mindful breath practices, and the men who practice the techniques onscreen clearly adore each other. Tapes that delve into male masturbation may be your best bet when looking for visual clues on ways men like to be touched and stimulated. Another from Joseph Kramer, *Evolutionary Masturbation: An Intimate Guide to Male Orgasm*, combines Tantra, sex toys (like cock rings and vibrators), and twenty masturbation techniques to show how to make men's masturbatory orgasms more intense. *Solo Male Ecstasy: An Intimate Guide to Self-Pleasure* is an instructional video on male masturbation that shows five men as they individually masturbate to orgasm, using a variety of techniques. The music is awful, but the men are nice-looking, and they discuss over forty genital massage techniques and ejaculatory control. Nothing advanced here, but it can augment your body of knowledge.

Recommended Reading

There's more erotica available now than ever, and a lot of it is of very high quality. You can find most anything you're looking for, if you know where to look, and there is no shortage of fellatio scenes. Erotica written by women provides a female perspective on sex and tends to concentrate on women's pleasure, which means that when fellatio is included it usually has the female character's sexual interests in mind. Lesbian erotica doesn't usually contain fellatio stories, but in some of the more modern, cutting-edge (and S/M) collections you can sometimes find women going down on a strap-on cock. In gay male erotica there's a lot of top-notch writing, and the stories are chock-full of fellatio scenes that portray the spectrum of scenarios; dirty, sweet, and everything in between. When straight men put pen to paper and write smut that contains fellatio, it tends to be either really good or transparent stroke material that verges on misogyny. Look for higher-quality anthologies and respected editors, authors, and publishers who produce reliably good books.

The *Best Women's Erotica* series is a combination heterosexual and lesbian anthology of short stories by and for women that comes out yearly and has an always-changing lineup of the best stories the genre produced in a given year. *Herotica* is a women-produced, women-focused anthology series that pioneered the for-women field. Both series contain explicit sex scenes, yet both have distinctively different flavors in their selections—thumb through them both and gauge your response. *Best American Erotica* comes out yearly, and it's where male and female authors of all orientations write erotica that is also of all orientations. *Black Lace* is a generally high-quality British imprint that features erotic novels written by women, and they occasionally put out collections of short stories that are worth picking up. *Black Lace* is heterosexually focused, though sometimes the novels do contain bisexual characters, and the fellatio in them is fantastic.

Best Lesbian Erotica is also a best-of yearly series but with only lesbian and dyke stories, and it smartly covers the spectrum and variations embodied in the many permutations of queer identity. Because it's true to the modern realities of lesbian sex, it occasionally includes strap-on fellatio scenes. *Best Bi Women's Erotica* is a yearly anthology series that features stories written by and for bisexual women. The stories contain women having sex with both men and women who identify as straight, lesbian, or bi, or don't identify as anything, and they introduce us to the sexual realities of bisexual women and the heat of bi sex; you get doses of fellatio here and there.

Following are my favorite fellatio short stories in contemporary erotica:

GAY MALE

"Below the Beltway," by Simon Sheppard. In *The Mammoth Book of Best New Erotica,* edited by Maxim Jakubowski (Carroll & Graf, 2001).

"The Color Khaki." In *See Dick Deconstruct,* by Ian Phillips (AttaGirl Press, 2001).

"Plaza del Sol," by Sean Wolfe. In *Friction 4,* edited by Jesse Grant (Alyson, 2001).

"Tiger Rag," by J. D. Ryan. In *Best Gay Erotica 2002,* edited by Richard Labonte (Cleis Press, 2002).

"Warm-up," by Matt Bernstein Sycamore. In *Best Gay Erotica 2001,* edited by Richard Labonte (Cleis Press, 2001).

HETEROSEXUAL/MIXED ORIENTATION

"Adventures in Dick Sucking," by Bree Coven. In *Best of the Best Lesbian Erotica,* edited by Tristan Taormino (Cleis Press, 2000).

"Do Me," by Lori Bryant Woolridge. In *Best Black Women's Erotica,* edited by Blanche Richardson (Cleis Press, 2001).

"Getting Dirty," by Erica Dumas. In *Sweet Life: Erotic Fantasies for Couples,* edited by Violet Blue (Cleis Press, 2001).

"On the Care and Feeding of White Boys," by R. Gay. In *Best Bisexual Women's Erotica*, edited by Cara Bruce (Cleis Press, 2001).

"What He Did," by Thomas Roche. In *Best American Erotica 1997*, edited by Susie Bright (Touchstone Books, 1997).

Sex Guides

Buying a sex guide is not very different from buying any other how-to guidebook—except that sex is a much more charged subject than, say, furniture upholstery. Though I'd be the first one to collect the *Time/Life Sex Series* (they'd be kept with no small amount of irony next to my ancient *Time/Life* books on plumbing and carpentry), it's doubtful that a book on sex could ever be so neatly packaged. Human sexuality doesn't fit into convenient cookbook categories, though many authors try to make it do so—and this is reflected in the sad state of the majority of sex guides that are available. Many guides commit the fatal crimes of being judgmental about preferences, fetishes, and orientations or being ill informed and containing inaccurate sex information. Good guides inform and don't sacrifice integrity for entertainment. I also don't like sex guides that lack substance and look like picture books combined with New Age poetry. What's worse are guides whose adolescent or self-indulgent attitude toward sex puts you off—be they written by men or women who must elevate or denigrate sexuality to make it palatable, or use instant-gratification sports terms. These antiquated attitudes about sex belong in a curio shop, not on your bookshelf.

When buying a sex guide, take a good look at it first. Do you like the tone, or is it too dry or condescending? See when it was published and if it's been revised recently (within the past five years, at the latest) to reflect current information. Try to look something up. Is the information easy to find? Does it have substance that you can use in a practical situation? Look up something nonmainstream such as S/M to see if the book has a judgmental attitude toward it—even if the practice isn't for you, the author's sex-negative attitude may hinder your exploration of other areas you might be interested in. And finally, does it have illustrations or pictures? You'll need them, so make sure they're there.

Guides for fellatio are pretty spotty; they tend to consist mostly of pictures and have the same techniques simply renamed to look more spiritual or cutesy than those in the author's last book, or just to look different. It's challenging to find books that will supplement your knowledge. Most overall sex guides have very tiny, sadly superficial treatments of fellatio—you get the feeling that they just didn't know what to say. But it is possible to find some great sex books to extend your sexual scope that will tie into the fellatio expertise you found in this book, and round out your sex life.

As general sex guides go, *The Good Vibrations Guide to Sex* by Cathy Winks and Anne Semans is a good cornerstone of any library; it's the most modern standard around for sex information, with a pleasure-centric approach, lots of sex practices that many people actually engage in but other guides won't include, and lots of sex toy info. *The Guide to Getting It On!* by Paul Joannides is hetero-centric and the tone is unbearably casual at times, but it's gigantic (over six hundred pages), has accurate information, and has sections not found in other tomes, such as a disabilities chapter. Every man who has sex with men should read *Men Like Us: The Complete GMHC Guide to Gay Men's Sexual,*

Physical, and Emotional Well-Being by Daniel Wolfe. It's an incredibly complete guide to virtually every aspect of gay male sexuality, and its approach and tone are wonderful.

There are many books on specific topics that relate to subjects covered in this book; they'll help you dig deep into what interests you. By far the best book out there on S/M and how to do it is Patrick Califia's *Sensuous Magic*. Califia mixes practical advice with scorchingly hot short stories to make a book that inspires and energizes on every level. *Come Hither* by Gloria Brame is a wonderful book about becoming interested in S/M and has unbeatable information on talking to your partner about it, or coping with your partner's wishes when they don't match up with yours. *Family Jewels* by Hardy Haberman explores the far reaches of cock and ball torture (CBT); and *The Ultimate Guide to Strap-On Sex* by Karlyn Lotney (a.k.a. Fairy Butch) tells all about strappin' it on and givin' it—to whomever you prefer.

Jack Morin's *The Erotic Mind* is older than most of the books I'm recommending, but it's very good; it explores the mind-set of having healthy, happy sex and digs deep into sex within long-term relationships. Folks who strive to become more sexually adventurous will want to read Carol Queen's *Exhibitionism for the Shy*, which gave me the courage and motivation to learn how to talk dirty in bed—you can learn exactly that in her book. *The Survivor's Guide to Sex* by Staci Haines is the first and best practical book for people who have survived trauma and/or abuse and want to have a fully present, satisfying and healthy sex life—it's indispensable. You can learn more about anal sex for women in the landmark book *The Ultimate Guide to Anal Sex for*

Women by Tristan Taormino, and the companion *Ultimate Guide to Anal Sex for Men* by Bill Brent is also highly recommended. *The Multi-Orgasmic Man: Sexual Secrets Every Man Should Know* by Mantak Chia and Douglas Abrams Arava explores multiple male orgasms and Tantric practices of orgasm without ejaculation. Heterosexually focused, it concentrates on combining breathing and the use of pressure points to achieve multiple orgasms in men. The book has a New Age tone throughout the text, which isn't for everyone—I find it distracting—but it is packed with much information.

Resources

Shopping for sex toys is an experience that can go one of two ways—success or frustration. Finding the toy you want takes both having an idea of what you might be looking for (or actually, looking to do), and finding a place that has your item. It's important to determine your intentions in advance; know what you'd like your toy to do, and have a specific item in mind. Or you might just be seeking inspiration by looking at toys, books, and videos. The other half of the equation is finding where to go, and knowing what they have there. If you're shopping in a store, it should be a comfortable place to shop; if a Web site, your privacy is important. And we hope that the folks running the shop know what they're doing and can answer questions about sex without giggling—or shrugging.

Most major cities have a selection of adult toy, book, and video shops that are somewhat (or even very) sleazy and uncomfortable to shop in, generally because they aren't clean or kept up in any visible way, and the customers and clerks don't seem to want to be seen there. My first trip into a woman-oriented sex toy store blew my mind—especially seeing all the other women and men shopping there—people of every stripe and persuasion, having fun buying vibrators and cock rings. Unfortunately these clean, well-lit places to shop for sex toys are found only in a few major cities. San Francisco (Good Vibrations), Seattle (Toys in Babeland), Austin (Forbidden Fruit), Boston (Grand Opening), New York (Toys in Babeland), Toronto (Come as You Are, Good for Her), and other cities have women-friendly sex toy shops, but many people choose to buy their products through mail order or the Internet. The privacy that the Internet affords has made it both easy and safe for everyone to try out new sexual ideas and explore new possibilities, and it puts sex toys within everyone's reach. However, the Internet can be dicey if you don't know the company's privacy policy (some companies sell your information to other parties), and it's more difficult to ask questions about the products.

Phone ordering is a little easier if you have a catalog, because you can ask questions, and ideally, get answers. Going into an actual store is really the best way to shop, and some people even go to the women-friendly shops to look at the toys, and then order from the privacy of their own homes. But since going into a local, friendly shop is not an option for everyone, here's a handy resource list, in alphabetical order.

Online and Mail Order

Adam and Eve

Mail-order catalog and Web site of toys, books, videos, DVDs, safer-sex supplies, and lingerie, with a hetero-sexual focus. The retail face of the mainstream adult industry; the site has a Spanish option, and they sell cus-tomer information to third parties.
P.O. Box 200, Carrboro, NC 27510
800 274 0333
919 644 1212
www.adameve.com

Blowfish

Mail-order catalog and Web site of toys, books, videos, DVDs, safer-sex supplies, S/M gear, comics, and maga-zines. They feature individual reviews of their products and a strict privacy policy.
P.O. Box 411290, San Francisco, CA 94141
800 325 2569
415 252 4340
www.blowfish.com

Blue Door

Buy or rent adult videos, with a nice selection helpfully divided into understandable sections. Videos are rated for excitement and entertainment and are individually reviewed by staff and customers. Strict privacy policy.
ETP Inc.
P.O. Box 64378, Sunnyvale, CA 94089
888 922 4387
www.bluedoor.com

Cetra Latex-Free Supplies

A product site for latex-free gear, mainly catering to the medical community (because so many medical professionals end up with latex allergies). Sells to individuals. Nice sitewide search.
888 LATEX NO
510 848 3345
www.latexfree.com

Condomania

Exhaustive site that sells virtually every condom under the sun, with fun facts, lots of condom information, and a helpful condom shopping guide.
1 800 9CONDOM
1 800 926 6366
www.condomania.com

Glyde Dams

Buy 'em here, by the dozen or in a party pack!
www.sheerglydedams.com

Good Vibrations

Promoting pleasure since 1977, Good Vibrations has a staff who are extensively trained and up-to-date on all things sex-related and are committed to dispensing accurate sex information about the products they sell. Mail-order catalog, Web site, and retail stores carry toys, books, videos, DVDs, safer-sex supplies, magazines, and comics. All products are individually selected and reviewed. The vibrators have volume and intensity ratings, and the Web site is loaded with sex information and even a magazine. Mail order is open 7:00 A.M. to 7:00 P.M., PST. Carol Queen is their staff sexologist. Strict

privacy policy. (For retail information, see the "Retail Stores" section below.)
938 Howard St., Ste. #101, San Francisco, CA 94103
800 289 8423
415 974 8980
www.goodvibes.com

Toys in Babeland

Web site, retail stores, and catalog of toys, books, videos, and safer-sex supplies. Women-owned and operated, but open to all orientations. Strict privacy policy. (For retail information, see the "Retail Stores" section below.)
800 658 9119
www.babeland.com

Xandria Collection

Mail-order catalog and Web site of toys, books, videos, DVDs, leather, and lingerie. Betty Dodson is on their advisory board. Xandria sells customer information to third parties.
165 Valley Dr., Brisbane, CA 94005
800 242 2823
415 468 3812
www.xandria.com

Retail Stores

A Woman's Touch

Feminist sex store offering toys, books, and safer-sex supplies. Their Web site has great advice columns.
600 Williamson St., Madison, WI 53703
608 250 1928
www.a-womans-touch.com

Come Again Erotic Emporium

Woman-owned store with toys, books, and lingerie; they also have a book and fetish catalog.
353 E. 53rd St., New York, NY 10022
212 308 9394

Eve's Garden

Woman-focused store and catalog of toys, books, and videos.
119 W. 57th St., Ste. #420, New York, NY 10019
800 848 3837
212 757 8651
www.evesgarden.com

Forbidden Fruit

Woman-owned and operated toy store/adult gift shop, fetish boutique, and body piercing/tattoo studio. A big supporter of the Austin S/M, fetish, safer-sex, and sex-positive communities.
Toy Store and Education Center
512 Neches St., Austin, TX 78701
512 478 8358

Fetish Boutique

108 North Loop Blvd., Austin, TX 78751
512 453 8090

Body Art Salon

513 E. Sixth St., Austin, TX 78701
512 476 4596
www.forbiddenfruit.com

Good Vibrations

Pioneering the woman-owned, woman-focused sex shop since 1977, this store has grown to employ and serve all communities and orientations with the mission of promoting pleasure and accurate sex information. Staff is meticulously trained, and their Education department serves staff and customers and does outreach to health organizations. Mail-order catalog, Web site, and retail stores carry toys, books, videos, DVDs, safer-sex supplies, magazines, and comics. All products are individually selected and reviewed, and they have ongoing After Hours classes in the stores. Carol Queen is their staff sexologist.

1210 Valencia St. San Francisco, CA 94110
415 974 8980

2504 San Pablo Ave., Berkeley, CA 94702
510 841 8987

Mail Order 800 289 8423
www.goodvibes.com
(See "Online and Mail Order" section for more mail order/Web info.)

Grand Opening!

Retail store, Web site, and mail-order catalog of toys, books, safer-sex supplies, and videos; store has classes and events, some taught and hosted by owner Kim Airs. 318 Harvard St., Ste. 32, Arcade Bldg., Coolidge Corner, Brookline, MA 02446
(Toll-free ordering) 877 731 2626
617 731 2626
www.grandopening.com

Passion Flower

Retail store of toys, books, lingerie, videos, and magazines. 4 Yosemite Ave., Oakland, CA 94611
510 601 7750

Pleasure Chest

Retail store, Web site, and catalog of novelties, toys, videos, and clothing.
7733 Santa Monica Blvd., West Hollywood, CA 90046
800 75 DILDO
323 650 1022
www.thepleasurechest.com

Purple Passion

Retail store and Web site of toys, books, videos, magazines, and fetish clothing and shoes, plus a full selection of S/M and bondage toys and accoutrements. Mainly geared toward BDSM shoppers. Many of their BDSM toys are handmade by craftswomen, and impact toys are rated for intensity.
242 W. 16th St., New York, NY 10011
212 807 0486
www.purplepassion.com

Rubber Tree

Retail shop for safer-sex goods.
4426 Burke Avenue No., Seattle, WA 98103
206 663 4750

Toys in Babeland

Retail store, Web site, and catalog of toys, books, videos, and safer-sex supplies. Women-owned and operated, but open to all orientations. They also have in-store educational workshops.
711 E. Pike St., Seattle, WA 98122
206 328 2914
94 Rivington St., New York, NY 10002
212 375 1701
(Mail order) 800 658 9119
www.babeland.com

Canadian Resources

Come As You Are

No visit to Toronto is complete without visiting this community-oriented worker-owned co-op retail store, and they also have a mail-order catalog and Web site. They have toys, books, videos, safer-sex supplies, and educational resources, especially resources for the disabled. Products are hand-picked and individually reviewed. Stores offer educational workshops. *Nous offrons des services limites en francais.*
701 Queen St. W., Toronto, ON, M6J 1E6, Canada
(Toll-free) 877 858 3160
416 504 7934
www.comeasyouare.com

Good For Her

Woman-focused retail store carries toys, books, videos, and erotic art; hosts sex workshops, all geared toward female pleasure. In addition to regular hours, store has women-only hours.
171 Harbord St., Toronto, ON, M5S 1H5, Canada
(Toll-free) 877 588 0900
416 588 0900
www.goodforher.com

Lovecraft

Retail stores and Web site offering toys, books, videos, and lingerie. Possibly the oldest women-owned sex shop in North America—open since 1972.
27 Yorkville Ave., Toronto, ON, M4W 1L1, Canada
416 923 7331

2200 Dundas St., East Mississauga, ON, L4X 2V3,
Canada
905 276 5772
(Toll-free) 877 923 7331
www.lovecraftsexshop.com

Womyn's Ware

Retail store, Web site, and catalog of toys, books, and
fetish gear, education- and woman-focused. Store hosts
sex seminars.
896 Commercial Dr., Vancouver, BC, V5L 3Y5, Canada
(Toll-free) 888 996 9273
www.womynsware.com

European Resources

SH!

A women's sex shop.
22 Coronet St. London N1, U.K.
Tel. (0171) 613 5458

Tiberius

Leather, Latex and Tools
Wien 7, Lindengassw 2, Austria
Tel. 43 1 522 040 74
www.tiberius.at
leather@tiberius.at

Safer-Sex Resources

American Social Health Association

P.O. Box 13827, Research Triangle Park, NC 27709
919 361 8400

Centers for Disease Control National AIDS Clearinghouse

P.O. Box 6003, Rockville, MD 20849
800 342 AIDS
www.cdcnac.com

National AIDS Hotline

800 342 2437

National STD Hotline

800 227 8922

Planned Parenthood

800 230 PLAN
www.ppfa.org

Safer Sex Page

www.safersex.org

San Francisco Sex Information

Sex information and referral switchboard that provides free, nonjudgmental, anonymous, accurate information. Monday through Friday 3:00 P.M. to 9:00 P.M. PST.
(Toll-free) 877 472 7374
415 989 SFSI
www.sfsi.org

Sex Education Classes and Workshops: Organizations

(For stores near you that offer sex education workshops and classes, see the "Retail Stores" section.)

Body Electric

School of healing arts dedicated to exploring the healing potential of erotic energy, with a holistic, mindful, and spiritual approach (open to all spiritual orientations). Classes for men and for women, mixed classes, retreats, and more, in Seattle, Oakland, New York, and Los Angeles.
6527-A Telegraph Ave., Oakland, CA 94609
510 653 1594
www.bodyelectric.org

The Fairy Butch Dynasty

Details magazine called Fairy Butch "the sexpert of a generation"; see why in her ongoing sex education classes in San Francisco.
www.fairybutch.com

San Francisco Sex Information

Sex information and referral switchboard that provides free, nonjudgmental, anonymous, accurate information. They offer a fifty-five-hour training course in all aspects of human sexuality; for more information, see their Web site.
(Toll-free) 877 472 7374
415 989 SFSI
www.sfsi.org

Society for Human Sexuality

Social and educational organization that offers lectures and programs in Seattle. They have a huge online library of sex resources.
PMB 1276, 1122 E. Pike St., Seattle, WA 98122
www.sexuality.org

Sex-Related Web Sites

AltSex

Information about all aspects of BDSM.
www.altsex.org

Betty Dodson

Betty's site—full of information.
www.bettydodson.com

Cleis Press

Cleis has published groundbreaking, informative, and controversial books about sex and politics since 1980. The publisher of this book, they also have a great Web site showcasing their latest erotica, all their sex guidebooks, and Midnight Editions, their incredible consciousness-raising human rights books.
www.cleispress.com

JackinWorld

Web site billed as the "ultimate male masturbation resource." Very informative.
www.jackinworld.com

Jane's Net

Reviewers cull oodles of sex-related and alternative lifestyle sites and list them with aplomb.
www.janesguide.com

Molly Kiely

This is the Web site of the artist whose cute and highly skilled illustrations grace the pages of this book. See more of her awesome work here—in full color!
www.mollykiely.com

Queer Net

Discussion lists galore for the lesbian, gay, bisexual, and transgender and S/M communities—you can even start your own.
www.queernet.org

Scarlet Letters

Webzine of articles, erotica, and more.
www.scarletletters.com

Scarleteen

Webzine of sex information geared toward teen women.
www.scarleteen.com

SIECUS (Sexuality Information and Education Council of the United States)

SIECUS is a national nonprofit organization that develops, collects, and disseminates information on sex, promotes sex education, and advocates individual choice.
130 W. 42nd St., Ste. 350, New York, NY 10036
212 819 9770
www.siecus.org

Tiny Nibbles

My very own site dedicated to all things relating to oral sex. Articles, orally fixated erotica, recommended reading, latest news, and more!
www.tinynibbles.com

Venus Or Vixen?

Read some smut! Fun-filled Webzine with articles, erotica, reviews, and more.
www.venusorvixen.com

References

Books

Alman, Isadora. *Doing It: Real People Having Really Good Sex*. Berkeley, CA: Conari Press, 2001.

Bechtel, Stefan, and Laurence Roy Stains. *Sex: A Man's Guide*. Emmaus, PA: Rodale Press, 1996.

Birch, Robert W. *Oral Caress: The Loving Guide to Exciting a Woman*. Howard, OH: PEC Publications, 1996.

Brame, Gloria. *Come Hither: A Common Sense Guide*. New York: A Fireside Book, Simon & Schuster, 2000.

Brent, Bill. *The Ultimate Guide to Anal Sex for Men*. San Francisco: Cleis Press, 2001.

Bruce, Cara, and Lisa Motanarelli, Ph. D. *The First Year: Hepatitis C*. New York: Marlowe and Co., 2002.

Califia, Patrick. *Sensuous Magic: A Guide for Adventurous Couples.* San Francisco: Cleis Press, 2001.

Chia, Mantak, and Douglas Abrams Arava. *The Multi-Orgasmic Man: Sexual Secrets Every Man Should Know.* San Francisco: Harper San Francisco, 1997.

Chia, Mantak, Maneewan Chia, Douglas Abrams, and Rachel Carlton Abrams, M.D. *The Multi-Orgasmic Couple.* San Francisco: Harper San Francisco, 2000.

Cox, Tracey. *Hot Sex: How to Do It.* New York: Bantam Books, Random House, 1999.

Gach, Michael Reed, Ph.D. *Acupressure for Lovers.* Bantam Books; Bantam Doubleday Dell Publishing Group, 1997.

Gilbaugh, James H., Jr., M.D. *Men's Private Parts: An Owner's Manual.* New York: Crown Trade Paperbacks, 1993.

Goldstone, Stephen E., M.D. *The Ins and Outs Of Gay Sex: A Medical Handbook For Men.* New York: Dell Publishing, Random House, 1999.

Haberman, Hardy. *Family Jewels: A Guide to Male Genital Play and Torment.* Emeryville, CA: Greenery Press, 2001.

Haines, Staci. *The Survivor's Guide to Sex.* San Francisco: Cleis Press, 1999.

Heiman, Julia, Ph.D., and Joseph LoPiccolo, Ph.D. *Becoming Orgasmic.* New York: Simon & Schuster, 1988.

Janus, S. S., and C. L. Janus. *The Janus Report on Sexual Behavior.* New York: Wiley, 1993.

Joannides, Paul. *The Guide to Getting It On!* Waldport, OR: Goofy Foot Press, 2000.

Lotney, Karlyn. *The Ultimate Guide to Strap-On Sex.* San Francisco: Cleis Press, 2000.

Masters, W. H., V. E. Johnson, and R. C. Kolodny. *Human Sexuality*. Boston: Little, Brown and Company, 1995.

———. *Masters and Johnson on Sex and Human Loving*. Boston: Little, Brown and Company, 1985.

Men's Fitness Magazine, with John and Beth Tomkiw. *Total Sex: Men's Fitness Magazine's Complete Guide to Everything Men Need to Know and Want To Know About Sex*. New York: Harper Perennial; Harper Collins Publishers, 1999.

Milsten, Richard, M.D., and Julian Slowinski, Psy. D. *The Sexual Male: Problems and Solutions* New York: W. W. Norton and Company, 1999.

Morin, Jack, Ph.D. *The Erotic Mind*. New York: Harper Perennial; Harper Collins Publishers, 1995.

Paget, Lou. *The Big O: Orgasms, How to Have Them, Give Them, and Keep Them Coming*. New York: Broadway Books, Random House, 2001.

———. *How to Be a Great Lover: Girlfriend-to-Girlfriend Time-Tested Techniques That Will Blow His Mind*. New York: Broadway Books, Random House, 1999.

Queen, Carol. *Exhibitionism for the Shy*. San Francisco: Down There Press, 1995.

Rodgers, Joann Ellison. *Sex: The Natural History of a Behavior*. New York: W. H. Freeman and Company, 2001.

Rogers, Ben R. and Joel Perry. *Going Down: The Instinct Guide to Oral Sex*. Los Angeles: Alyson Publications, 2002.

Sheiner, Marcy. *Sex for the Clueless*. New York: Citadel Press, 2001.

Stubbs, Kenneth Ray, Ph.D. *Erotic Passions*. Tucson, AZ: Secret Garden Publishing, 2000.

————. *Male Erotic Massage.* Tucson, AZ: Secret Garden Publishing, 1999.

Taormino, Tristan. *The Ultimate Guide to Anal Sex for Women.* San Francisco: Cleis Press, 1998.

Walker, Mitch. *Men Loving Men: A Gay Sex Guide and Consciousness Book.* San Francisco: Gay Sunshine Press, 1997.

Winks, Cathy, and Anne Semans. *The Good Vibrations Guide to the G-Spot.* San Francisco: Down There Press, 1998.

————. *The New Good Vibrations Guide to Sex,* 2nd ed. San Francisco: Cleis Press, 1997.

Wolfe, Daniel. *Men Like Us: The GMHC Complete Guide to Gay Men's Sexual, Physical, and Emotional Well-Being.* New York: Ballantine Books, 2000.

Zilbergeld, Bernie, Ph. D. *The New Male Sexuality: The Truth About Men, Sex and Pleasure.* New York: Bantam Books, 1999.

Videos

Britton, Patti, Ph.D., F.A.A.C.S. *The Complete Guide to Oral Lovemaking*. Sexual Enrichment Series; Pacific Media Entertainment, 1997.

Hartley, Nina. *Nina Hartley's Guide to Fellatio*. Adam and Eve Productions, 1994.

———. *Nina Hartley's Advanced Guide to Oral Sex*. Adam and Eve Productions, 1998.

———. *Nina Hartley's Making Love to Men*. Adam and Eve Productions, 2000.

Kessler Medical Rehabilitation Research and Education Corporation. *Sexuality Reborn*. Kessler Medical Rehabilitation Research and Education Corporation, 1993.

Kramer, Joseph. *Fire on the Mountain: An Intimate Guide to Male Genital Massage*. Joseph Kramer/The Body Electric School, 1993.

———. *Evolutionary Masturbation: An Intimate Guide to Male Orgasm*. Joseph Kramer/The Body Electric School, 1996.

———. *Uranus: Self Anal Massage for Men*. Joseph Kramer/The Body Electric School, 1996.

Sinclair Institute. *Better Oral Sex Techniques*. Better Sex Video Series; Sinclair Institute, 1997.

Zaffuto, Dr. Anthony A. *Solo Male Ecstasy: An Intimate Guide to Self-Pleasure*. 1996.

About the Author

VIOLET BLUE is senior copywriter at Good Vibrations where she writes book and video reviews, which has her watching an awful lot of porn, and reading virtually everything imaginable about sex. She is a sex columnist and a sex educator. She is the editor of *Sweet Life: Erotic Fantasies for Couples*, and the author of two books on oral sex, *The Ultimate Guide to Cunnilingus* and *The Ultimate Guide to Fellatio*. Visit her web site about all things oral, tinynibbles.com. When not on the job Violet pursues her other passions, mostly working on giant machines in Survival Research Laboratories, drinking tasty red wines, and searching for the perfect chocolate croissant.